T0175965

UNDERSTANDING THE

NURSING PROCESS

IN A CHANGING CARE ENVIRONMENT

NOTICE

Medicine and nursing are ever-changing sciences. As new research and clinical experience broaden our knowledge, changes in treatment and drug therapy are required. The authors and the publisher of this work have checked with sources believed to be reliable in their efforts to provide information that is complete and generally in accord with the standards accepted at the time of publication. However, in view of the possibility of human error or changes in medical sciences, neither the authors, nor the publisher, nor any other party who has been involved in the preparation or publication of this work warrants that the information contained herein is in every respect accurate or complete, and they are not responsible for any errors or omissions or for the results obtained from use of such information. Readers are encouraged to confirm the information contained herein with other sources. For example and in particular, readers are advised to check the product information sheet included in the package of each drug they plan to administer to be certain that the information contained in this book is accurate and that changes have not been made in the recommended dose or in the contraindications for administration. This recommendation is of particular importance in connection with new or infrequently used drugs.

Sixth Edition

UNDERSTANDING THE
NURSING PROCESS

IN A CHANGING CARE ENVIRONMENT

Mary Ellen Murray, Ph.D., R.N.

Assistant Professor
School of Nursing
University of Wisconsin–Madison

Leslie D. Atkinson, R.N., M.S.N.

Nursing Program
Normandale Community College
Bloomington, Minnesota

Illustrated by Mark Atkinson

McGraw-Hill

Health Professions Division

New York   St. Louis   San Francisco   Auckland   Bogotá   Caracas
Lisbon   London   Madrid   Mexico City   Milan   Montreal   New Delhi
San Juan   Singapore   Sydney   Tokyo   Toronto

Mcgraw-Hill

A Division of The McGraw-Hill Companies

Understanding The Nursing Process, Sixth Edition
Copyright © 2000, 1994 by The McGraw-Hill Companies, Inc. All rights reserved. Printed in the United States of America. Except as permitted under the United States Copyright Act of 1976, no part of this publication may be reproduced or distributed in any form or by any means, or stored in a data base or retrieval system, without the prior written permission of the publisher.

6 7 8 9 10 QVSQVS 20 19 18 17 16 15

ISBN 0-07-135078-0

This book was set in Times Roman by Better Graphics, Inc. The editors were John Dolan and Catherine Wenz; the production supervisor was Richard Ruzycka; the editing supervisor was Karen Edmonson; the text and cover were designed by Marsha Cohen, Parallelogram.
R. R. Donnelley & Sons was printer and binder.

This book is printed on acid-free paper.

Cataloging-in Publication Data is on file for this title at the Library of Congress.

Dedication
To Peter
To Craig

CONTENTS

PREFACE   xiii

CHAPTER ONE

Introduction to the Nursing Process   1

Nursing: What Is It? / 1
The Nursing Process: What Is It? / 2
Why Is the Nursing Process Important? / 5
Critical Thinking in Nursing / 8
    Critical Thinking, Problem Solving, and Clinical Judgment / 9
    Critical Thinking and the Nursing Process / 9
    Components of Critical Thinking for Clinical Judgment / 10
    Who Are Critical Thinkers? / 11
        Characteristics of Critical Thinkers / 11
Culturally Competent Nursing Care / 12
    Culture: Mine, Ours, and Theirs / 12
    Cultural Concepts / 14
        Communication / 14
        Space / 14
        Social Organization / 15
        Time / 15
        Environmental Control / 16
        Biological Variations / 16
    Awareness of Own Culture: What Is the Dominant American
       Culture Like? / 16
        Communication / 17
        Space / 17
        Social Organization / 17
        Time / 18
        Environmental Control / 18
        Biological Variations / 18

Nursing Process: The Managed Care Environment / 18
Changes Leading to Managed Care / 18
The Impact of Managed Care on Nursing Practice / 19
What Does It Mean to Be Fiscally Accountable in Your
Nursing Practice? / 22
Cost-Effective Nursing Care / 23

CHAPTER TWO

Assessment   25

Data Collection / 26
Data Collection Format / 26
Maslow's Basic Need Framework / 27
Henderson's Component's of Nursing Care / 29
Gordon's Functional Health Patterns / 30
NANDA's Human Response Patterns / 30
Nursing Theories / 30
Human Growth and Development / 31
Data Collection Skills / 33
Observation / 34
Interview / 35
Examination / 40
Medical Record Review / 42
Critical Thinking for Assessment / 43
Prompts for Critical Thinking during Assessment / 44
Critical Thinking Practice Exercises during Assessment / 44
Culturally Competent Nursing Care during Assessment / 48
Prompts for Culturally Competent Nursing Care
during Assessment / 49
Assessment: The Managed Care Environment / 51
Case Management Plan / 51
Assessment of Health Care Resources / 53
Summary / 54
Practice Exercise / 54
Answers to Exercise on Assessment / 55
Case Study: Assessment / 56
#1 Nursing Assessment: Preoperative Orthopedic
Surgery Clinic / 57
#2 Nursing Assessment: First Day Surgery
Center: 6 A.M. / 59
#3 Nursing Assessment: Postoperative Orthopedic
Patient Care Unit / 61
#4 Nursing Assessment: Home Health Care Agency / 61

CHAPTER THREE

Diagnosis   65

Data Analysis / 66
Problem Identification / 68
Formulating the Nursing Diagnosis / 77
    Types of Nursing Diagnoses / 78
        Actual Nursing Diagnoses / 78
        Risk Nursing Diagnoses / 79
        Possible Nursing Diagnoses / 79
    Collaborative Problems / 81
    Writing Nursing Diagnoses / 82
        Actual Nursing Diagnoses / 82
        At-Risk/High Risk Nursing Diagnoses / 83
        Possible Nursing Diagnoses / 83
    Validating Nursing Diagnoses / 84
Critical Thinking for Diagnosis / 85
    Prompts for Critical Thinking during Diagnosis / 85
Culturally Competent Nursing Care during Diagnosis / 86
    Prompts for Culturally Competent Nursing Care
        during Diagnosis / 86
Nursing Diagnosis: The Managed Care Environment / 88
Summary / 90
Practice Exercise / 90
Answers to Exercise on Nursing Diagnosis / 91
Case Study: Nursing Diagnosis / 92
    #1 Nursing Diagnosis: Preoperative Orthopedic
        Surgery Clinic / 92
    #2 Nursing Diagnosis: First Day Surgery Center: 6 A.M. / 93
    #3 Nursing Diagnosis: Postoperative Orthopedic
        Patient Care Unit / 94
    #4 Nursing Diagnosis: Home Health Care Agency / 95

CHAPTER FOUR

Outcome Identification   99

Activities in the Outcome Identification Phase / 100
Setting Priorities / 100
    Guidelines for Setting Priorities / 100
Establishing Outcomes / 102
    Why Is an Outcome Statement Needed? / 103

Components of an Outcome Statement / 104
Patient Behavior / 104
Criterion of Performance / 105
Conditions / 106
Time Frame / 106
Guidelines for Writing Outcome Statements / 111
Classification of Nursing Outcomes / 115
Critical Thinking for Outcome Identification / 117
Prompts for Critical Thinking during Outcome
Identification / 118
Culturally Competent Nursing Care during Outcome
Identification / 118
Prompts for Culturally Competent Nursing Care during
Outcome Identification / 119
Patient Outcomes: The Managed Care Environment / 119
Summary / 121
Practice Exercise / 121
Answers to Exercise on Outcome Statements / 122
Case Study: Outcome Identification / 124
#1 Patient Outcomes: Preoperative Orthopedic
Surgery Clinic / 124
#2 Patient Outcomes: First Day Surgery Center: 6 A.M. / 125
#3 Patient Outcomes: Postoperative Orthopedic Patient
Care Unit / 125
#4 Patient Outcomes: Home Health Care Agency / 126

CHAPTER FIVE

Planning   127

Types of Nursing Interventions / 128
Environmental Management / 128
Physician-Initiated and -Ordered Interventions / 129
Nurse-Initiated and Physician-Ordered Interventions / 130
Nurse-Initiated and -Ordered Interventions / 130
Rationale for Nursing Interventions / 132
Problem Solving and Selecting Interventions / 134
Patient Teaching: An Intervention Strategy / 137
Classification of Nursing Interventions / 143
Critical Thinking for Planning / 144
Prompts for Critical Thinking during Planning / 148
Culturally Competent Nursing Care during Planning / 148
Prompts for Culturally Competent Nursing Care
during Planning / 149
Planning: The Managed Care Environment / 150

Summary / 151
Case Study: Planning / 152
   #1 Planning: Preoperative Orthopedic Surgery Clinic / 152
   #2 Planning: First Day Surgery Center: 6 A.M. / 153
   #3 Planning: Postoperative Orthopedic Patient Care Unit / 155
   #4 Planning: Home Health Care Agency / 157

CHAPTER SIX

Implementation   159

Validating the Care Plan / 159
Documenting the Nursing Care Plan / 161
Giving and Documenting Nursing Care / 163
Continuing Data Collection / 164
Critical Thinking for Implementation / 165
   Prompts for Critical Thinking during Implementation / 165
Culturally Competent Nursing Care during Implementation / 166
   Prompts for Culturally Competent Nursing Care during
      Implementation / 166
Implementation: The Managed Care Environment / 166
Summary / 169
Critical Pathway / 169

CHAPTER SEVEN

Evaluation   183

Documenting Responses to Interventions / 183
Evaluating the Effectiveness of Interventions / 184
Evaluation of Outcome Achievement / 185
   Patient Participation and Evaluation / 185
   Writing an Evaluative Statement / 186
Review of the Nursing Care Plan / 189
   Reassessment / 189
   Review of Nursing Diagnoses / 190
   Review of Outcomes and Replanning / 191
   Review of Implementation / 193
Critical Thinking for Evaluation / 194
   Prompts for Critical Thinking during Evaluation / 194
Culturally Competent Nursing Care during Evaluation / 195
   Prompts for Culturally Competent Nursing Care
      during Evaluation / 197
Evaluation: The Managed Care Environment / 197
Summary / 198

Case Study: Evaluation / 200
#1 Evaluation: Preoperative Orthopedic Surgery Clinic / 200
#2 Evaluation: First Day Surgery Center: 7 A.M. / 201
#3 Evaluation: Postoperative Orthopedic Patient Care Unit / 202
#4 Evaluation: Home Health Care Agency / 204

BIBLIOGRAPHY   207

APPENDIX A

Sample Nursing Care Plans   211

Nursing Care Plan #1. Middle Adult / 211
Critical/Clinical Pathway—CHF (Congestive Heart Failure) / 218
   by Elizabeth Clark, RN, MSN
Nursing Care Plan #2. Senior Adult / 222
   by Tom Olson, RN, PhD

APPENDIX B

Web Sites   231

General Nursing Web Sites / 231
General Cultural Web Sites / 231
Specific Cultural References / 231

INDEX   235

APPENDIX C

Nursing Diagnosis Pocketbook (In Book Sleeve)

PREFACE

As nursing and health care enter the new century, we believe that several key changes will dominate. These concepts have been incorporated into our sixth edition of *Understanding the Nursing Process in a Changing Care Environment*. This is a book for students starting their nursing programs, and so the ideas are presented at a basic level as they relate to the nursing process and beginning patient care. These ideas include

- The importance of critical thinking skills for clinical practice
- The managed care environment with increasing standardization of patient care
- The need for nurses to be involved in the economic side of care and for this to be reflected in their practice.
- The increasing multiculturalism of society
- The increasing percentage of patients who will be elderly

When the first edition of *Understanding the Nursing Process* was published in 1980, there were four phases in the process: assess, plan, implement, and evaluate. The new edition has six phases, with a new separate chapter for outcome identification. In 1980, the North American Nursing Diagnosis Association (NANDA) had not yet been formed and nursing diagnoses were created by the individual nurse. There were no lists of approved nursing diagnoses with definitions and defining characteristics. Patient outcomes were a new idea to most nurses. Most practicing nurses had not been taught about the nursing process as part of their formal education. This does not mean that expert clinical judgment was lacking; it was just less formalized in its teaching and documentation.

MANAGED CARE, COSTS, AND STANDARDIZATION OF PATIENT CARE

The last half of the 1990s has seen an increasing amount of standardization of care planning and documentation of the nursing process. This standardization is part of the managed care environment. This edition reflects the emphasis on

managed care with a section describing its application in each step of the nursing process. With managed care, clinical/critical pathways are replacing traditional nurse-developed care plans based on assessments of individual patients. Patients are put on the appropriate pathway on the basis of the medical diagnosis, and the nurse helps the patient meet predetermined outcomes to move through the system to discharge in a timely, cost-effective manner. The need to contain health costs is the driving force in managed care, and we believe that nursing education in the future must include the economic side of care. We have incorporated pathways in this edition to complement the traditional care-planning activities and emphasize the unique patient and the need to individualize standard critical/clinical pathways.

Further standardization of the care-planning components of the nursing process comes from nurse researchers in Iowa. The Iowa Interventions Project published the second edition of *Nursing Interventions Classification (NIC)* in 1996. A total of 433 interventions are defined and classified with a set of specific activities for nurses to use in implementing each of the general interventions. In addition, *Nursing Outcomes Classification (NOC)* has been published with specific indicators nurses can use to evaluate the effectiveness of interventions. The NANDA nursing diagnoses and the NIC and NOC texts are all linked to standardize language and usage for care planning. We congratulate them on their work and have included examples in several chapters.

THE NURSING PROCESS AND CRITICAL THINKING

Today the concept of critical thinking is viewed as crucial to high-quality nursing care. Does this mean that nurses in the past were not critical thinkers? Of course not. But the concept has become more clearly defined, and programs in nursing are now teaching critical thinking instead of hoping it will develop in their graduates if they are given enough knowledge and clinical experience. We have included sections in each chapter to reflect this focus. We believe that critical thinking activities are embedded in each phase of the nursing process. We also believe that the nursing process is cyclical in nature rather than linear and forms the "thinking framework" for clinical decision making as a nurse. Prompts for critical thinking are offered to the reader in each chapter, with exercises in critical thinking included in the chapter on assessment.

We continue to believe students in nursing must learn the nursing process and care plan development from the beginning of their education. Each step in the nursing process and care plan development is explained at a level appropriate to a beginning nursing student. Clinically, students may be using critical pathways and not developing individual care plans, but "thinking like a nurse" is dependent on learning the process of disciplined thinking resulting from the use of the nursing process. The product, whether it is a traditional care plan, a

critical pathway, or whatever form may evolve in the future, is based on this fundamental, structured form of clinical reasoning.

INCREASING CULTURAL DIVERSITY

The changing demographics of the U.S. population point to increasing diversity in the cultural and racial backround of our patients over the next few decades. Currently, approximately 75% of the population of the United States is European-American, but by the year 2050, the prediction is that one in two Americans will be African, Asian, or Hispanic in racial/ethnic backround. This important demographic change will affect who gives and receives health care. This edition includes a section on culturally competent care in each chapter. Prompts for culturally competent care in each step of the nursing process may help students think about areas to assess or adaptations to consider when giving care to patients from a wide variety of cultures. A Web site reference page in Appendix B is available as an information source on various cultures.

AGING OF SOCIETY

In addition to cultural factors, age factors will change patient demographics. More than 80% of patients in hospitals will be over 65 years of age. The elderly are less able to go from acute-care hospital settings to independent home discharge, especially with the shortened length of stay most insurance providers are willing to cover in the hospital. Because of this, patients will be moved from one setting to the next until home discharge is possible. To reflect this trend, our end-of-chapter care plans have been changed to show the progress of an older adult through the system, from a preoperative teaching session, to first day surgery admission, to a postoperative hospital setting, and finally to a home health care agency.

The American Nurses Association (ANA) revised the Standards of Clinical Nursing Practice in 1998 to reflect some of the changes in practice. The original version, published in 1973, was built around the steps in the nursing process, and the activity of outcome identification was added in the 1991 version. The six activities of the nursing process as presented in the 1998 *Standards of Clinical Nursing Practice* are reflected in the chapter divisions of this edition, with a separate chapter for outcome identification. The term *patient* is used instead of *client* in the 1998 *Standards of Clinical Nursing Practice*. We have always favored the use of this term to reflect the recipients of nursing care, whether individuals, families, groups, or communities. In addition, the term *family* is used in the broadest sense in this edition to reflect the changed terminology in the ANA Standards.

We again wish to thank our friends, and family who have put up with us during this revision and our colleagues and students who keep asking questions and questioning the status quo as we move into the new millennium. We celebrate this profession of nursing in all its diversity, asking, Now what? and Why not?

Once again, the order of authorship of this text was decided by the flip of a coin and reflects our continued happy collaboration.

Mary Ellen (Knedle) Murray
Leslie D. Atkinson

ACKNOWLEDGMENTS

A special thank you to the following individuals who contributed to the sixth edition of *Understanding the Nursing Process in a Changing Care Environment*

Tom Olson, RN, PhD
University of Hawaii at Manoa
Senior Adult Care Plan and its most current revision

Elizabeth Clark, RN, MS, PCRN
Cardiovascular Clinical Nurse Specialist
North Memorial Medical Center, Minneapolis, Minnesota
Review of the Middle Adult Care Plan and her original clinical pathway

Ronnie Peterson, RN, MSN
Chairperson, Interdisciplinary/Multicultural Patient Care Team
University of Wisconsin Hospital and Clinics, Madison, Wisconsin

Barbara A. Liegel, RN, MSN, CS
Director of Home Health Agency
University of Wisconsin Hospital and Clinics, Madison, Wisconsin

Judith E. Broad, RN, PhD
Senior Vice President, Nursing and Social Work
University of Wisconsin Hospital and Clinics, Madison, Wisconsin

Heidi Norwick, BSN, RN
Orthopedic Nurse Case Manager
University of Wisconsin Hospital and Clinics, Madison, Wisconsin

Sharon J. Trimborn, RN, PhD
Assistant Vice President of Nursing
University of Wisconsin Hospital and Clinics, Madison, Wisconsin

Jessica E. Murray, BA, for her typing expertise

Mark Atkinson for his past and current illustrations

UNDERSTANDING THE

NURSING
PROCESS

IN A CHANGING CARE
ENVIRONMENT

CHAPTER 1

Introduction to the Nursing Process

NURSING: WHAT IS IT?

Nursing has been described in many different ways by many different leaders and theorists in the field. What is unique about nursing? What service does nursing provide to patients that no other health care profession provides? The founder of modern nursing, Florence Nightingale, in her *Notes on Nursing* published in 1859, defined nursing as having "charge of the personal health of somebody" and went on to say that "what nursing has to do . . . is to put the patient in the best possible condition for nature to act upon him." The American Nurses Association (ANA), which is the professional organization for nurses in the United States, defined nursing in 1980 and reaffirmed that definition in 1995. That definition describes the scope of nursing practice:

> Nursing is the diagnosis and treatment of human responses to actual or potential health problems.

(Reprinted with permission from American Nurses Association, *Nursing—A Social Policy Statement*, © 1995 American Nurses Publishing, American Nurses Foundation/American Nurses Association, Washington, D.C.)

This means, for example, that nursing is not responsible for diagnosing and treating cancer; the physician does that. Nursing is primarily responsible for diagnosing and treating a patient's response to the cancer and medical treatment, such as inadequate nutrition, nausea, altered self-esteem, anxiety, and pain. Nursing is involved in aspects of the medical treatment, as in giving a patient prescribed medication or treatments, but the primary focus of nursing is the patient's response to health-related problems. It is also important to understand that the term *patient* is used to describe a recipient of nursing care in the broadest possible sense. Sometimes the patient is a single individual, but a family or a community can be the focus of nursing care.

In 1995, the ANA also recognized four essential elements of nursing practice that definitions of nursing increasingly include:

1. Nursing includes attention to the full range of human experience and responses to health and illness, without restriction to a problem-focused orientation.
2. Nursing integrates objective data with the knowledge gained from an understanding of the patient's subjective experience.
3. Nursing includes the application of scientific knowledge to the processes of diagnosis and treatment.
4. Nursing provides a caring relationship that facilitates health and healing.

(Reprinted with permission from American Nurses Association, *Nursing—A Social Policy Statement*, © 1995 American Nurses Publishing, American Nurses Foundation/American Nurses Association, Washington, D.C.)

THE NURSING PROCESS: WHAT IS IT?

The nursing process is the way one thinks like a nurse. This process is the foundation, the essential, enduring skill that has characterized nursing from the beginning of the profession. Through the years, the nursing process has changed and evolved, growing in clarity and scope.

The nursing process is divided into six steps:

1. ASSESSMENT:
What brought you to the hospital?
Let me have a look at that.
I'd like to listen to your lungs.
Please describe how you are feeling.
When did the problem start?

2. DIAGNOSIS:
What is the problem?
What is the cause?
How do I know it?
Is there additional information that I need to verify my thinking?

3. OUTCOME IDENTIFICATION:
How do I know the problem is better?
This is where we hope you will be by tonight, by tomorrow, by discharge.
What are the goals the patient (and family) and I have agreed to?
What are the results I want to achieve from the nursing interventions?
Do we have enough resources (time, energy, money, supplies) to accomplish the goals?

4. PLANNING:
What can I do about it?
What is most important?
What do I want to happen and by when?

5. IMPLEMENTATION:
Move into action.
Carry out the plan.

6. EVALUATION:
Did it work? Why or why not?
Is the problem solved, or do I need to try again?
Revise the plan based on new information.

While these steps are an oversimplification, every nurse has already had much practice with the problem-solving or scientific process. Consider the college chemistry course that is required for all nurses. The students are asked to observe and examine the properties of different chemicals and to perform a series of planned experiments utilizing those substances. Hopefully, the student, through the use of this scientific problem-solving process, has discovered the solution to the question of how certain chemicals react. These steps are essentially the same as those used in the nursing process.

The nurse uses these six steps in *every* interaction with a patient, no matter how brief the contact. Expert nurses have mastered this process to such a high degree that they are unaware of using the separate steps in the process. In fact, in describing expert nursing practice, Benner states:

It is not possible to recapture the explicit formal steps, the mental processes that go into experts' capacity to make rapid patient assessments. . . . To assume that it is possible to capture all the steps in nursing practice is to assume that nursing is procedural rather than holistic. Attempts may be made to model or make explicit all the steps that go into a nursing decision, but experts do not actually make decisions in this elemental, procedural way. They do not build up their conclusions, element by element; rather, they grasp the whole. Even when they try to give detailed accounts of the elements that went into their decisions, essential elements are left out. (Benner, 1984, pp. 42–43)

This process is the foundation, the essential, enduring skill that has characterized nursing from the beginning of the profession . . .

Assess: *"A careful nurse will keep a constant watch over her sick. . . . The feet and legs should be examined by the hand from time to time."*
                                                                                      p. 11
"For it may safely be said, not that the habit of ready and correct observation will by itself make us useful nurses, but that without it we shall be useless with all our devotion."
                                                                                      p. 63

(*continued on p. 4*)

(continued)

Diagnose: *"I will tell you what was the cause of this hospital pyaemia being in that large private house. . . . It was that sewer from an ill-placed sink."*   *p. 17*

Identify outcome: *"In surgical wards, one duty of every nurse is certainly* prevention. *Fever, or hospital gangrene, or pyaemia or purulent discharge of some kind . . ."*   *p. 71*
"Whatever a patient can *do for himself, it is better . . . for him to do for himself."*   *p. 22*

Plan: *"There are five essential points in securing the health of houses: pure air, pure water, efficient drainage, cleanliness, lights."*   *p. 14*
"Keep the air he breathes as pure as the external air without chilling him."   *p. 8*

Implement: *"To be 'in charge' is certainly not only to carry out the proper measures but to see that everyone else does so too; to see that no one either willfully or ignorantly thwarts or prevents such measures."*
                                                                       p. 24
"Never allow a patient to be waked, intentionally or accidentally. . . . If he is roused out of his first sleep, he is almost certain to have no more sleep."
                                                                       p. 25

Evaluate: *"Surely you can learn at least to judge with the eye how much an oz. of food is, how much an oz. of liquid. You will find this helps your observation and memory very much. You will then say to yourself, 'A. took about an oz. of his meat today'; 'B. took three times in 24 hours about 1/4 pint of beef tea,' instead of saying, 'B. has taken nothing all day,' or 'I gave A. his dinner as usual.'*   *p. 64*

Adapted from: Florence Nightingale, *Notes on Nursing, What It Is and What It Is Not.* From an unabridged facsimile of the first edition printed in London, 1859. Reproduced by offset in 1946. Philadelphia: Edward Stern & Company, Inc.

It is not that experts do not use the nursing process but rather that they are so skilled in using it that it has become integrated into their thinking.

A more easily understood example of Benner's hypothesis is the skill of driving a car. Somewhere around age 16, most people (to the dismay and consternation of parental figures) begin a driver's education course. We all memorize and complete a driver's assessment before turning on the ignition: First, walk around the car to check for obstacles and tire safety; then adjust mirrors, adjust driver seat height and distance from pedals, lock doors, adjust seat belt, check fuel gauge, and so forth. Finally, the driver can start the car and go. However, after a few years of experience, the driver just does these things automati-

cally and probably would be unable to relate the steps that were so conscious only a short time ago. This book is to nursing what the driver's education manual is to driving.

One outcome of the use of the nursing process is a plan of care for the patient. This plan of care may look very different from institution to institution. One hospital may choose a handwritten plan on a form devised for that purpose. Another hospital may use preprinted or computerized plans. But each of these plans contains the essential components of planned patient care.

WHY IS THE NURSING PROCESS IMPORTANT?

Two driving forces emerged in the 1990s that had a major impact on clinical nursing practice: the *emphasis on quality* and the *emergence of managed care* as a dominant force in health care financing. The demand for quality comes from accreditation agencies, consumers of health care, and payers of health care. In each setting in which nurses work, requirements are set by accrediting agencies that mandate that quality improvement programs be ongoing and that the results of those programs be measured and evaluated.

Consumers of health care are becoming increasingly aware that all health care is not of equal quality. Consider that a recent Internet search for the phrase *quality in health care* showed 4,617,754 hits. One relevant address is http://www.ncqa.org, the home page of the National Committee for Quality Assurance (NCQA). The savvy consumer may read, on-line, the NCQA consumer brochure, *Choosing Quality*.

Finally, payers of health care services such as insurance companies and managed health care plans are beginning to compete not only on the basis of cost but also on the basis of the quality of care provided. Many health maintenance organizations (HMOs) are publishing their quality ratings and patient satisfaction data as public information.

Nurses continually seek ways to improve their practice and the satisfaction of the patients they serve. If nursing is to survive the competitive challenges of the new millennium, it must continue to provide a high-quality service that patients value. The nursing process provides a tool for nurses in all settings to use to continually evaluate and improve the quality of nursing care. One example of a quality-improvement project might be a situation in which nurses observed that patients being admitted on the morning of surgery did not receive thorough preoperative instruction and did not understand how to use their pain control machines. Nurses working on this project could use the steps of the nursing process to complete an assessment of the problem and define its causes. Next, they would determine the outcomes they hoped to achieve by making changes in clinical practice. They would develop a plan and, at a predetermined time, evaluate the results of their practice change.

The second major trend in the 1990s, the emphasis on cost containment, affected all areas of health care. Because hospitals are the most expensive part

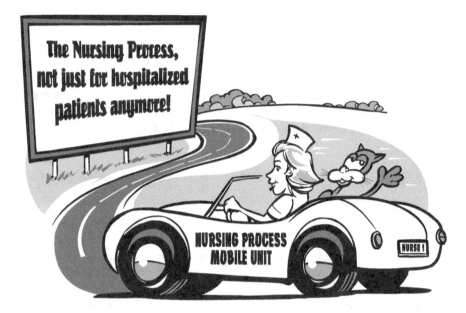

The Nursing Process, not just for hospitalized patients anymore!

NURSING PROCESS MOBILE UNIT

NURSE 1

FIGURE 1-1.   On the road with the nursing process!

of the health care system, they were most strongly affected. Most noticeable to nurses was the decreased length of stay for patients. All the teaching and discharge planning for patients had to be compressed into shorter periods. However, the upside to this was the concurrent growth in home health nursing. After hospitalization, many patients were referred to home health agencies for continuing care. The use of the nursing process will help the nurse continually assess and reassess the patient's response to illness and then plan appropriate care in any setting for illness care or health promotion.

The American Nurses Association has published *Standards of Clinical Nursing Practice* (1998). Standards used in this sense define the responsibilities of all registered nurses engaged in clinical practice regardless of the setting (see Table 1-1). These standards list the nurse's responsibility to the public. The standards hold the nurse accountable for the use of the nursing process. It is important that students understand that the standards do not mandate that the use of the process result in a specific form of care plan. That degree of specificity is a function of the clinical setting in which the nurse is working. But the standards do require evidence of this critical thinking process, which all nurses use to plan and evaluate care.

In addition to meeting the Standards of Nursing Clinical Practice, there are other advantages for nurses who become skilled in the use of the nursing process:

TABLE 1-1   STANDARDS OF CLINICAL NURSING PRACTICE

Standard I.	**Assessment** The Nurse Collects Patient Health Data.
Standard II.	**Diagnosis** The Nurse Analyzes the Assessment Data in Determining Diagnoses.
Standard III.	**Outcome Identification** The Nurse Identifies Expected Outcomes Individualized to the Patient.
Standard IV.	**Planning** The Nurse Develops a Plan of Care That Prescribes Interventions to Attain Expected Outcomes.
Standard V.	**Implementation** The Nurse Implements the Interventions Identified in the Plan of Care.
Standard VI.	**Evaluation** The Nurse Evaluates the Patient's Progress toward Attainment of Outcomes.

Source: Reprinted with permission from American Nurses Association, *Standards of Clinical Nursing Practice*, 2nd edition, © 1998 American Nurses Publishing, American Nurses Foundation/ American Nurses Association, Washington, D.C.

1. *Graduation from an Accredited School of Nursing.* All types of nursing programs (diploma, associate degree, and baccalaureate) require students to have a basic competency in the use of the nursing process upon graduation.

2. *Confidence.* Care plans resulting from the nursing process let the student or the staff nurse know specifically what problems the patient has, what goals are important for the patient, and how and when they might best be accomplished.

3. *Job Satisfaction.* Good care plans can save time, energy, and the frustration generated by trial-and-error nursing from staff members and students whose efforts remain uncoordinated. Coordinating a patient's nursing care through a care plan greatly increases the chances of achieving a successful resolution of health problems. The nurse and student should feel a real sense of accomplishment and professional pride when outcomes in a care plan are met.

4. *Professional Growth.* Care plans provide an opportunity to share knowledge and experience. Collaboration with colleagues in formulating a nursing care plan will add to an inexperienced nurse's clinical skill. Later, during the process of evaluation, the nurse or student receives the feedback necessary to decide how effective the nursing care plan was in dealing with the patient's problems. If the plan worked well, the nurse may use a similar approach in the future. If it failed, the nurse can explore possible reasons for the undesirable results with the patient, other staff members, other students, an instructor, or a clinical nurse specialist.

5. *Aid in Staff Assignments.* Care plans assist nurse managers, team leaders, and nursing instructors in making the most appropriate patient assignments by showing the degree of complexity involved in an individual patient's care plan. Could an aide follow the care plan and provide good care, or is a professional nurse required? Could students work with this patient, or is the plan of care beyond their knowledge and experience? What aspects of nursing care can be safely delegated?

6. *Employment in a Nationally Accredited Hospital.* Hospitals are approved by a national commission to help ensure that patients receive quality care. The following statements are taken directly from the accreditation manual for hospitals and are a requirement for accreditation.

P.E. 1. Each patient's physical, psychological, and social status are assessed.

P.E. 2.3. Significant change in a patient's condition results in reassessment.

P.E. 3. Staff members integrate the information from various assessments of the patient to identify and assign priorities to his or her care needs.

P.E. 4.3. A registered nurse assesses the patient's needs for nursing care in all settings where nursing care is provided.

Tx. 1.3. Patient's progress is periodically evaluated against care goals and the plan of care and when indicated, the plan or goals are revised.

CC. 6.1. The discharge process provides for continuing care based upon the patient's assessed needs at the time of discharge.

(Used with permission. 1999 Hospital Accreditation Standards. Joint Commission on the Accreditation of Healthcare Organizations.)

CRITICAL THINKING IN NURSING

Critical thinking has been defined in a variety of ways in the literature. Common themes run through most of these definitions.

- It is a *reasoning* or thinking *process.*
- It is *disciplined* rather than random or accidental.
- It is *reflective* in that it looks back at what has been and "rethinks" the situation.
- It is *purposeful.* Some of the purposes for critical thinking include the following:
  Searching for meaning
  Producing and evaluating ideas and making plans
  Deciding what to believe and do; making competent decisions
  Seeking ways to improve things regardless of whether a problem exists
  Preventing and resolving problems by considering many options
  Developing one's potential; teaching oneself
  Improving efficiency

Critical thinkers consider personal biases and beliefs, integrate new information and actual outcomes, and rethink the situation, trying to find a better way of doing things.

Critical Thinking In Nursing

is disciplined, purposeful, reflective reasoning focused on finding meaning and improving the current situation.

Based on these themes and purposes from the literature, *critical thinking* in nursing can be defined as purposeful, disciplined, reflective reasoning focused on finding meaning, deciding what to believe and do, and improving the current situation. It is based on evidence (data) rather than personal values, biases, or guesswork. It is thinking "out of the box" by people who say, "What if . . . " or "Why not . . . " and "Now what?" It is not easy, and it is not always safe because new ideas and change can be frightening. Doing things "the way we have always done it" is safe. It is easy. It is not creative. It does not require learning and applying new information or knowledge. But critical thinking is the kind of thinking needed to help our patients and their families adapt and improve their health in a constantly changing world. Nurses who do not think critically are part of the problem. What kind of a nurse do you want to be?

Critical Thinking, Problem Solving, and Clinical Judgment

Critical thinking is related to *problem solving* but is more than that. Problem solving begins when a negative situation—a problem—is identified and ends when that problem is resolved. Critical thinking may begin with positive events and outcomes as the nurse tries to figure out why things went so well and how this improvement could be repeated in similar or new situations. Critical thinking goes beyond problem solving. It is like the Windows version compared with the old DOS operating system for computers: It lets you do much more. *Clinical judgment* is critical thinking in the clinical area. It involves knowledge, skill and experience, ethics, reflection, and problem solving as the nurse applies the nursing process to determine with the patient what the patient's health needs are both now and in the future and how best to meet those needs in a direct care setting.

Critical Thinking and the Nursing Process

Critical thinking is used during each step of the nursing process and is part of the process viewed as a whole. The nursing process is the framework around

which the nurse does critical thinking. Without critical thinking, the steps in the nursing process would be followed like a recipe, step by step, with no creativity. It would be a narrow, potentially biased focus that would overlook subtle patient concerns and be limited to obvious problems. All patients would be treated in a standard way, with no consideration of the uniqueness of this patient, in this situation, with these types of strengths and weaknesses. Uninspired and minimally safe is how the nursing process would seem without critical thinking occurring during each step. Critical thinking and the nursing process combine to result in the most complete, effective, and efficient nursing care for each unique patient.

Components of Critical Thinking for Clinical Judgment

There are several components of critical thinking, all of which fall into three areas:

- Cognitive skills (thinking)
- Affective skills (feelings and beliefs)
- Personality traits

We all possess some critical thinking ability in areas where we have knowledge, skill, and experience. With practice, the ability to do critical thinking in new areas can be developed, but it will take work. In the clinical setting, the ability to think critically and develop good clinical judgment is based on the integration of five components (modified with permission from Kataoka-Yahiro and Saylor, 1994):

Good Clinical Judgment In Nursing $=$

Knowledge $+$ Clinical Experience $+$ Reasoning Skills Using Nursing Process $+$ Attitudes $+$ Standards

- *Knowledge* of information from nursing and related courses: "book learning"
- *Experience* giving patient care and making clinical decisions: "hands-on learning"
- *Reasoning skills* that give the framework for thinking: use of the nursing process
- *Attitudes* that motivate internally so that you "gotta wanna know": curiosity, confidence that you can, courage to try to go against the status quo, perseverance, willingness to admit you were wrong
- *Standards* of the nursing profession specifically and more general standards of clear thinking and fairness: doing the best job you can and measuring it against standards such as completeness, accuracy, and logic

The ability to think critically develops over time as a student in nursing gains knowledge, skill, and experience in a variety of patient care settings. A graduate nurse begins the career of nursing as a generalist but also as a novice. With time and work, the nurse will become a critical thinker making sound clinical judgments that safeguard and improve patient care in a focused area of nursing.

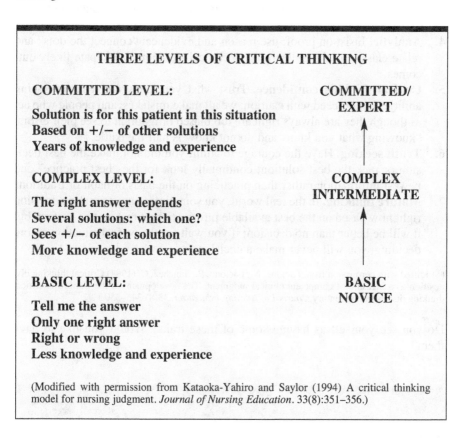

THREE LEVELS OF CRITICAL THINKING

COMMITTED LEVEL:

Solution is for this patient in this situation
Based on +/− of other solutions
Years of knowledge and experience

COMMITTED/ EXPERT

COMPLEX LEVEL:

The right answer depends
Several solutions: which one?
Sees +/− of each solution
More knowledge and experience

COMPLEX INTERMEDIATE

BASIC LEVEL:

Tell me the answer
Only one right answer
Right or wrong
Less knowledge and experience

BASIC NOVICE

(Modified with permission from Kataoka-Yahiro and Saylor (1994) A critical thinking model for nursing judgment. *Journal of Nursing Education.* 33(8):351–356.)

Who Are Critical Thinkers?

Critical thinkers have many similar personality traits. They ask questions and try to understand different beliefs and viewpoints. They are open to different ways of doing things but insist on evidence to prove that a change is better. These characteristics can be developed. Work and study with people around you who have these traits. Use them as role models; ask them what they are thinking and what things they considered in making a decision. Select their best processes and approaches and adapt them to your style.

CHARACTERISTICS OF CRITICAL THINKERS.   Characteristics of a critical thinker include the following:

1. **Inquisitive.** "You've got to want to know" new ideas, knowledge, and skills.
2. **Systematic.** Get a system and use it consistently even if you think you know the answer.
3. **Open-minded.** My way of thinking and believing is only one of many, all of which have advantages and disadvantages and are right or wrong only in context of culture, families, communities, and unique individuals and situations.
4. **Analytic.** Insist on proof; use reason and evidence; "connect the dots" and relate classroom theory learning to clinical situations; anticipate likely outcomes.
5. **Critical thinking confidence.** Trust what you know and your reasoning abilities but proceed with caution; we all make mistakes, and people who act as though they are always right are too biased or ignorant to see their errors; "knowing what you know and do not know is half the battle."
6. **Truth seeking.** Have the courage to admit you did not make the best decision or pick the best solution; continually look for the "best practice" and newest information rather than practicing on the basis of habit or tradition.
7. **Mature thinking.** In the real world, you sometimes have to make a decision right now based on the best available information; it may not be perfect, but it will be better than no decision; if you wait for the perfect situation before deciding, you will never make a decision.

(Modified with permission from Facione, N., Facione, P., Sanchez, C. (1994) Critical thinking disposition as a measure of competent clinical judgment: The development of the California critical thinking disposition inventory. *Journal of Nursing Education*, 33(8):345–350.)

Do you see yourself as having some of these traits? Would you like to have them?

CULTURALLY COMPETENT NURSING CARE

Culture: Mine, Ours, and Theirs

In the beginning we have our family and our neighborhood, and we learn the answers to many questions: Who am I? What language do I speak? What do I believe in? How should I act? What genetic traits, both positive and negative, run in my family? What does my family do when I am sick to make me better? What traditions do we have for births? For deaths?

As adults, we became nurses and associated with health care professionals and learned the answers to many questions: What is a nurse? What do all those medical terms and abbreviations mean? What values does the profession believe in? What behavior is expected of nurses in a care setting? What can we do? What can't we do? What are the positives and negatives of professional nursing

as a career? What do standards of practice guide us to do for health problems? What specific nursing interventions and treatments are best for patients and specific problems? What is our role at birth? At death?

As we become culturally sensitive individuals and nurses, we see our patients as individuals within their cultures and learn the answers to many questions: Who are they? What language do they speak? What are their cultures' general values and beliefs? What does this patient believe in? How do patients think they should act? What genetic traits, both positive and negative, are in their ethnic/racial background? What do they think is causing their health problem, and what do they think will make it better? What family or cultural treatments have they been using? Which of these treatments do they believe are important to continue? What behaviors or traditions are important for them to continue while receiving nursing care? For births? For deaths?

We all are very ethnocentric as children. *Ethnocentrism* is the belief that one's own cultural beliefs and values are "right." We are not even aware of other cultures; thus, there is only one culture—ours. As we mature, we may become aware of other cultures with different values, beliefs, and behaviors, but ours is still viewed as the "best," the only acceptable culture. For example, our tradition of laying babies down for sleep on their tummies so that they do not choke is the right way to do it. Our mothers and their mothers taught this to us. However, some other cultures have always put their babies to sleep on their backs. They are wrong. We must teach them the right way. This is ethnocentrism. As it turns out, tummy lying is a risk factor for sudden infant death syndrome (SIDS), and the United States launched a massive effort beginning in 1992 to reverse this cultural tradition; our SIDS death rate has decreased markedly because of it. Oops!

As future nurses, you will be giving care to an increasingly diverse patient population. In the United States the dominant culture (75%) is European-American or Anglo-Saxon. By the year 2050, the estimate is that one in two Americans will be African, Asian, or Hispanic in racial/ethnic background. Culture defines how a group of people think, believe, and behave. It must be incorporated into the delivery of health care if that care is to be acceptable, meaningful, and respectful of multicultural patients.

Cultures are

- Learned (nonphysical, socially inherited traits)
- Transmitted from generation to generation
- A guide to living life and viewing the world
- A means of providing comfort and security to their members through practices and traditions
- A set of shared traditions, language, beliefs, values, and behaviors
- Part of an individual's beliefs about health and illness, prevention and treatment
- Often shared ethnicity/race; may have physical variations and disease risk factors

The goal of nursing is to provide culturally sensitive, individualized care that blends a patient's cultural beliefs with Western health care practices in a harmonious, complementary way. This is not always easy. The term frequently applied to this type of nursing is *culturally competent nursing care*. There are several components to culturally competent care. Awareness of one's own cultural background is important, as is awareness that Western medicine is one of many health care cultures in the world. Knowledge and respect for other cultures are crucial if your goal is to provide competent nursing care for patients of various cultures. Being nondiscriminatory and being nonjudgmental are ways of showing acceptance and support for patients' values and beliefs. Cultural competence in many cultures is an unrealistic expectation. It is expected, however, that you will become culturally competent with cultures you routinely encounter in your practice, just as you become technically competent in dealing with patients who have similar health problems and treatments. Regardless of your knowledge of a culture, always assess each individual in a manner that considers cultural aspects and the uniqueness of the individual. See the Web sites for various cultures in Appendix B.

Components of Culturally Competent Nursing Care =

Awareness and Knowledge	+ Communication Skills	+ Attitude of Respect	+ Nonjudg-mental
• Own Culture	• Verbal		
• Patient's Culture	• Nonverbal		
• Nursing Culture	• Interpreters		

Cultural Concepts

There are six concepts, common to all cultural groups (Giger and Davidhizar, 1991), that nurses can consider as they learn to provide more culturally appropriate nursing care.

COMMUNICATION.   Communication is the means by which culture is transmitted and preserved. One's culture directs how one's feelings and thoughts are expressed, both verbally and nonverbally, and often creates a barrier if the nurse and the patient are from different cultures. The language itself may be understood by both people, but cultural orientation may affect their understanding of the message. Nonverbal expressions are crucial to understanding the message. Gestures, facial expressions, eye contact, and body language can give words a different meaning when viewed from two different cultures.

SPACE.   People's comfort level is affected by the area that surrounds them: their personal space. We feel most secure in our own personal space surrounded

with familiar things. We become uneasy when our personal space is invaded. We respond with behavior such as pushing back a chair, stepping back, or turning away. "Don't crowd me" and "Get out of my face" are slang expressions that reflect this need for personal space. Touching is involved in this concept, with some cultures having high touch norms and some having low norms. There are certainly individual variations, but people in the same cultural group tend to act similarly in relation to spatial needs.

SOCIAL ORGANIZATION.   The family is a basic unit of all societies, but roles and structure vary among cultures. A family is two or more individuals who come from the same or different biologically related groups. Families can be one generation or several generations with people connected by marriage, birth, adoption, or mutual agreement. The head of the household may be identified by cultural tradition based on sex, age, or mutual consent. The organizational structure of the family determines who makes major decisions about health care. The nurse needs to understand the structure to provide information and seek approval from the appropriate family or religious leader regarding the care of one of the members. Groups of people held together by similar beliefs and interests make up the social organization of a culture. The nursing profession is an example of a social organization within the health care culture.

TIME.   One's culture provides a time orientation from which to view and relate to the world. A year, a month, and a week may all have different lengths compared to the Western 365 days in a year, 30 to 31 days in a month, and 7 days in a week. For example, a "week" may vary from several days to 20 days or more, depending on the culture. The idea of being "on time" has different meaning to various cultural groups. A woman from Africa told me that in her culture, being several hours late based on the Western time concept is still "on time" and would not be considered late.

Some cultures are future-oriented, which means that the future is a key factor in a person's present behavior. There is a fairly clear view of an expected future if one engages in this type of behavior today. American and Western medicine is future-oriented. A future orientation to health and disease is essential to preventive medicine. People with a future orientation say, "I'll get back to you," "We can do it later," "You need to save for retirement," "Get a good education," "Eat right, exercise, and quit smoking to prevent heart disease."

Cultures with a present orientation have little concern for the future or the past. The main focus of living is on meeting today's needs. A causal relationship between today's behavior and an expected future outcome is difficult for people in present-oriented cultures to understand. The harder individuals have to work to meet basic survival needs on a daily basis, the more likely they are to be present-oriented. The only real time is the here and now; the promise of future benefits from current efforts is a foreign concept. The Hmong culture, for example, views time in the present, and therefore, follow-up care often is neglected. People who have a present orientation say, "Do it now," "You'll never come this way again," "Seize the moment," "It's now or never." They may forget about appointments and change plans on an impulse.

Cultures that have a past orientation view the past and traditions as most important and the future as too distant to worry about. Change is very difficult for people with a past time orientation regardless of the reported future benefits of the change. Many Asian cultures place a high value on the past and on tradition. They may place great faith in traditional treatments for illness. People who have a past orientation to time say, "We've always done it this way. Why change now?" "You can't teach an old dog new tricks," "Tradition tells us to do this."

Western medicine and the nursing profession are future-oriented and view time as very important. Nurses say, "Do not waste time," "Give those medications on time," "Patients should be bathed and groomed by 10 A.M." (regardless of whether the patient has the same time frame). Treatments are done on time and on a set schedule such as 8–12–4–8. The underlying cultural concept is that if this activity is done today, this outcome will be reached tomorrow. This works well for patients who are also future-oriented but less well for present-oriented patients and least well for past-oriented patients.

ENVIRONMENTAL CONTROL.   This concept relates to who or what is in charge of an individual's destiny: the individual, God, evil forces, or natural events. Does the culture view control as coming from the individual or coming from external forces? Is health viewed as something the individual controls, something the environment and nature control, or a balance between those forces? Is illness an imbalance in an individual's spiritual, physical, and social world, or is it caused by a bacteria or virus? Health-related behavior and treatment of injury or illness are determined by how the culture empowers the environment and the individual.

BIOLOGICAL VARIATIONS.   People in different racial and cultural groups may have some biological differences. Body size and shape, eyelids, teeth, skin color, reactions to drugs, and the risk for certain illnesses or diseases can all vary with race. Hypertension and sickle cell disease are more common in the African-American population, skin cancer is more common in European-Americans, and diabetes is more common in the Native American population.

Awareness of Own Culture: What Is the Dominant American Culture Like?

Generalizations about any culture tend to be partly true and partly false for specific individuals within that culture. Stereotyping people within a culture misses this individuality. *Stereotyping* people means that once you identify the culture and have some general knowledge about behavior, values, and biological variations in that culture, you assume that all individuals in that culture follow those behaviors and values. A culturally competent nurse assesses each unique individual on the basis of general knowledge of the culture to better understand this individual, in this situation, at this time. To see how generalizations work, the dominant culture in the United States will be examined based on the six concepts that are present in all cultures. Do all of these generalizations apply to you? Do

any? Would you want your health care to be based only on these generalizations about the dominant U.S. culture?

COMMUNICATION

- English is the dominant language
- Name: children take father's last name; one or more given names; middle name may relate to mother's family (maiden name)
- Value freedom of expression to communicate beliefs
- Less likely to verbalize or express feelings than some other cultures
- Low-touch culture
  Hugs and embraces among close family, intimates
  Women do more hugging and touching than men
  Pat on shoulder indicates friendship
  Long touch interpreted as sexual
  Value firm handshake as sign of good character and strength
- Facial nonverbal meaning
  Value eye contact; sign of strength, interest, attentiveness, and honesty
  Lack of eye contact interpreted as rudeness, inattentiveness, guilt, embarrassment
  Cold stare, rolling the eyes are signs of disagreement or disapproval
  Tight lips are interpreted as a sign of anger
- Other nonverbal behavior
  Palms up can mean "I'll go along with something even if I disagree"
  Thumbs up means "I'm all for it; great idea"; thumbs down means "I'm against it"
  Leaning toward a person conveys attention to what the other person is saying
  Less touching of children for soothing, holding, and play than some other cultures

SPACE

- Americans, Canadians, and British desire more space than most cultures
  0–18″ = intimate zone; reserved for people who feel close; touch can occur
  18″–3 ft = personal zone; used with friends; touch can occur
  3–6 ft = social or public zone; for impersonal business, coworkers
- Sleeping: parents separate from child versus group sleeping arrangements
- Personal possessions important versus shared possessions
- Dislike any infringement on their space, possessions, or actions
- Materialistic: collect lots of "stuff," especially technical equipment; throw away and buy new
- People's bedrooms are their own space for their own things versus shared

SOCIAL ORGANIZATION

- Value equal gender roles and rights
- Value youth and beauty: culture does not respect or value the wisdom of the elderly
- Very individualistic versus conforming
- Dominant family form is the nuclear family (a small group consisting of parent or parents and nonadult children living in a single household)

- Value competition and assertiveness and are achievement-oriented rather than cooperative and conforming to group norms
- Generous and helpful in crisis
- Legal system derived from English common law; political system from France and England
- Health care institutions based on Anglo-American values and practices

TIME
- Future-oriented
- Values related to future orientation: thrift, education, saving for retirement
- Time is money (life run by clock); being on time or early is expected and valued
- Value saving time and using time more efficiently
- Expect services and appointments to be "on time"; being forced to wait (10–15 minutes) may cause anger and be viewed as poor service

ENVIRONMENTAL CONTROL
- Believe in self-determination; individual control over environment; value individualism and self-reliance; independence and freedom
- Biomedical model of health care
- Reliance on scientific facts and numbers as the way of knowing what is true; reliance on technology
- Take many pills/medications to treat or prevent health problems; less reliance on heat/cold, relaxation, massage, ceremony, balance of spiritual with biological
- Doing is related to success; value being active

BIOLOGICAL VARIATIONS
- Anglo-American (Caucasians who trace their heritage largely from Europe)
- Tend to be taller than other races (as do African-Americans); Asian-Americans shorter
- Dominant blood type is A+ and O+; Rh-negative blood more common in whites
- Type 1 diabetes more common in Anglo-American men; type 2 diabetes more common in nonwhites and women
- Breast cancer and skin cancer more common
- Tend to be stoic about pain

NURSING PROCESS: THE MANAGED CARE ENVIRONMENT

Changes Leading to Managed Care

In 1996, national expenditures for health care topped a trillion dollars. In the 1950s and 1960s, health care costs in the United States grew out of control under

the fee for service (FFS) payment system. This system meant that the patient, the hospital, or the provider (doctors, clinics, etc.) presented a bill and the insurance company paid it, usually without any question. There was no incentive to be cost-efficient. In fact, the opposite was true. Under the FFS system, there was an incentive to do more because each service was billed to the patient or insurance company and was paid promptly. Patients were given multiple diagnostic tests and procedures and actually convalesced in the hospital, staying until they were independent in their care. It was not unusual for a nurse to care for several hospitalized patients who were taking showers and being up ad lib while awaiting a gastrointestinal (GI) x-ray series. Each part of the series would be done on sequential days: day 1, an upper GI x-ray; day 2, a lower GI x-ray; day 3, a proctoscopy. Today, with almost no exceptions, all these procedures are routinely done on an outpatient basis as a cost-saving measure.

In 1965, Medicare became law as part of the Social Security Act. The purpose of Medicare is to provide health insurance to the elderly, most of whose health insurance was provided by their employers and therefore stopped after retirement. Medicare costs were uncontrolled until 1983, when the federal government introduced diagnostic-related groupings (DRGs). DRGs are a classification system that groups patients according to medical diagnoses, average length of hospitalization, age, and so on. Under this system, it is assumed that each DRG can be effectively treated by using a certain amount of resources (nursing, drugs, treatments, surgeries, and therapies). The federal government determines in advance that a fixed amount of money will be paid for each patient whose disease or surgical procedure is classified within a given DRG. If a hospital can keep the costs of care below the DRG Medicare reimbursement, it makes a profit: The hospital can keep the difference between the actual cost of care and the Medicare payment. However, if the cost of treating the patient is more than the DRG payment, the hospital loses money. Medicare expenditures nationally rose from $7.7 billion in 1970 to $187 billion in 1995.

The Impact of Managed Care on Nursing Practice

Managed care developed in response to out-of-control health care costs. In fact, the managed care industry has been successful in decreasing the rate of increase of health care expenditures. Few nurses are able to define managed care or discuss how it affects their clinical practice. To understand what is meant by managed care, it is helpful to think of managed care as both a process and a system of reimbursement for health care.

As a process, managed care is defined as patients receiving the right care, by the right provider, in the right amount, at the right time, in the right place. In this sense, nurses have always managed patient care. When a patient is in the hospital, it is the nurse who assures that the patient has the correct preparation for a test, that diagnostic procedures are scheduled in the appropriate sequence, and that treatments occur as ordered and are discontinued when they no longer are needed. For example, when first admitted, a patient may require a very

expensive special bed to prevent pressure ulcers. As the patient's status improves and he or she becomes ambulatory, the nurse discontinues the unneeded special bed as a cost-saving measure. Another nurse may be caring for a patient who is scheduled to have physical therapy treatments twice a day. When it is 1 P.M. and the patient has not yet had a treatment, the nurse calls the physical therapy department to investigate the cause of the problem and determine a schedule. This is the process of managing patient care.

Managed care as a system of reimbursement includes patients, health care providers, and insurance companies. Most often the patient has health care insurance that is fully or partially paid for by an employer. The employer contracts for health insurance for employees from a health care provider as a benefit of employment. Within this system, there are guidelines to control the use of health care services and subsequently the cost of those services. Most managed care arrangements require that a patient select a primary care provider (PCP). Traditionally, the PCP has been a physician, but now the PCP frequently is a nurse practitioner. The PCP is responsible for the health care of the patient, and all referrals to specialists must come from the PCP. Those referrals must be consistent with certain guidelines to prevent overuse of costly specialty services and treatments. An example of a guideline might be that a patient will be referred to a specialist for one consultation visit. All the following visits for treatments must be preapproved or the insurance company will not pay for them. In this way, the managed care company maintains control over the use and cost of services.

Another way in which managed care companies attempt to control costs is through the use of nurse case managers. In a nursing case management model, both medical care and nursing care are combined into one complementary plan with the goal of providing quality care that is cost-effective. Multidisciplinary health care providers collaborate to design this plan of care for use on all patients with the same clinical problem. An example might be a case management plan for patients who have had a myocardial infarction (MI), DRG 122. Experienced nurses and physicians know that there are certain predictable problems and needs that most patients with this diagnosis will develop. Caregivers identify daily outcomes for MI patients that are most likely to progress them to discharge in a timely manner. Similarly, certain diagnostic procedures and medical treatments are common to this medical diagnosis. They are included in the case management plan as standard physician orders used for all patients with this DRG. Expert nurses also can predict that certain nursing diagnoses will occur frequently in these patients. Those nursing diagnoses are selected for inclusion in the case management plan. Nursing experts also have learned which nursing interventions are likely to be most effective in resolving or preventing the high-frequency nursing diagnoses. These are the interventions selected for the plan. This plan may be documented as a *critical pathway, clinical pathway,* or *care pathway*. The essential component of the plan is that it specifies all the care the patient is to receive on a time schedule, with clinical outcomes for each time period. In this system, the nurse caring for the patient is still responsible for the assessment of the individual patient, but the critical pathway is designed to be appropriate for the majority of patients in a particular category. The nurse must

still adapt the plan of care for an individual patient who may have additional problems or may recover faster or slower than anticipated in the case management plan. Table 1-2 compares the steps of the nursing process to a case management plan.

Nurse case managers are responsible for assuring that each patient has a plan of care and that resources are used in a cost-effective manner. Some nurse case managers work for insurance companies, coordinating the care of a group of patients across all the settings in which patients receive care. They are often the first-line decision makers for determining which services will be approved for payment by the insurance company. Other nurse case managers work in hospitals or community settings. They usually have no authority to approve payment but are responsible for developing case management plans that use health care resources for the maximum benefit of the patient and the cost-effectiveness of the organization.

TABLE 1-2   A COMPARISON OF THE STEPS OF THE NURSING PROCESS AND THE CASE MANAGEMENT PLAN

	Nursing Process	Case Management Plan
Assessment	Individual patient data	Pooled patient data base
Diagnosis	Individualized, based on nursing assessment of one patient	High-frequency diagnoses from pooled database of the same DRG
Outcome Identification	Agreement between nurse and patient regarding end result of care	Outcomes reflect usual expectation of interventions for this clinical patient population
Planning	Interventions selected by one nurse based on abilities of one individual nurse for needs of one individual patient; timing of interventions independently selected by one nurse	Interventions selected by multidisciplinary experts; time line reflects usual or anticipated recovery time line
Implementation	Focus on giving care	Focus on meeting time-defined outcomes and on coordination of care
Evaluation	Document evaluation of patient outcomes or progress toward outcomes	Document variance from expected outcomes, interventions to get patient back on time line of outcomes leading to discharge

For most of the history of modern nursing, probably until the beginning of managed care, nurses and most physicians abdicated any responsibility for the financial aspects of clinical practice. They sought to give "total patient care" and "quality patient care" without considering the costs to patients or their employing organizations. Today practicing nursing without an awareness of costs is irresponsible and does not give patients the very best care. Consider the case of Mrs. Jones, whose only insurance is Medicare. The physician writes an order for a very expensive medication that Mrs. Jones will need on a long-term basis. If the nurse does not understand the Medicare system, the patient may go home and not have the money to pay for the medication. Frequently this is the case with elderly patients on a fixed income. A responsible nurse understands that Medicare does not pay for prescriptions and may do further assessment to determine whether Mrs. Jones can afford this medication. The nurse also may consult with the physician to see if a less expensive drug can be substituted or may request a social service consultation to secure funding.

What Does It Mean to Be Fiscally Accountable In Your Nursing Practice?

To be fiscally accountable means that a nurse uses the most cost-efficient resources to maximize the health care benefit to the patient. A nurse in a managed care environment needs to understand the costs of care and differing reimbursement practices. This will affect the development of the plan of care. A beginning nurse should not mistakenly interpret this to mean that a patient who cannot pay for care will not receive care. Clinical decisions should not be based on the patient's ability to pay. Rather, the health care team needs to explore other treatment plans or find other resources to care for this patient. For example, the newer drug Zofran costs $28.79 per pill, whereas Compazine costs $6.47 per pill. Both control nausea and vomiting. A fiscally accountable physician or nurse uses Compazine unless it doesn't work or is contraindicated for this patient (Snyder Pharmacy, Minneapolis, MN, 4/99). In this new environment, nurses must be willing to talk about the costs of care with patients. Patients have a right to understand the costs of care and make decisions about alternative plans. Patients are consumers and purchasers of health care and may make decisions that differ from those that professionals might make for them.

From another perspective, nurses need to examine their clinical practice for cost efficiencies. The most costly item that staff nurses control is the allocation of their time. Understanding this leads nurses to examine which aspects of care must be done by a professional nurse and which may be delegated safely to less-trained personnel. Another example involves the timeliness of discharge planning. Nurses must think about discharge planning from the first meeting with the patient, not waiting until the patient is ready to leave the hospital or be transferred to another care setting. A final example considers the use of supplies in patient care. Cost-conscious practice requires that the nurse use what is needed but not bring duplicates of all supplies into the patient's room. Once supplies are

in a patient's room, they are considered contaminated and cannot be used for another patient. It also may be possible to select supplies that meet the need of the patient but are less expensive, such as different types of dressings or intravenous (IV) tubing. It is also important to charge out supplies accurately so that they are billed correctly to the patient. If the charges are not correctly billed, the hospital must absorb the costs as a loss. Hospitals that operate at a loss do not stay open long.

Cost-Effective Nursing Care

Cost containment has changed nursing practice in many ways. An intermittent IV is flushed with normal saline rather than heparin to keep it patent. Saline is less expensive, and studies show that it works as well as a heparin flush. Betadine is no longer used routinely to treat a newborn's umbilical cord. Alcohol three times a day is just as effective and is cheaper.

Nurses strive to balance quality patient care and cost containment. In the Standards of Professional Practice, the ANA describes competent levels of behavior in the professional nurse role. Standard VIII addresses resource utilization.

STANDARD VIII. RESOURCE UTILIZATION

The Nurse Considers Factors Related to Safety, Effectiveness and Cost in Planning and Delivering Patient Care.

Reprinted with permission from American Nurses Association, *Standards of Clinical Nursing Practice*, 2nd edition, © 1998 American Nurses Publishing, American Nurses Foundation/American Nurses Association, Washington D.C.

In defining the measurement criteria for this standard, the ANA indicates that it is a responsibility of the nurse to consider safety, effectiveness, availability, and cost when selecting from two or more interventions that would result in the same patient outcome. The ANA also states that it is the responsibility of the nurse to help patients and families become informed consumers about the cost, risks, and benefits of treatment and care.

What is best for the patient may not always match the patient care guidelines or interventions identified on critical pathways. Nurses have a dual responsibility to patients and to their employing institutions. Some situations may create conflict for nurses who understand these competing demands. Nurses have always been patient advocates. This ethical responsibility always guides decision making and clinical care. Often, the best care is cost-effective. Consider the patient who is rating her pain as 7 to 8 on a 10-point scale after bowel resection surgery. This patient is unable to use an incentive spirometer, walk in the hall, or do resistance exercises in bed. The inability to do these activities may

increase the length of stay and lead to complications. The patient who receives more-aggressive pain management is able to participate actively, and this results in a more rapid recovery. The initially more costly intervention of aggressive pain management is actually cost-effective. Table 1-3 will help you consider your fiscal responsibility for nursing practice both for your patients and for your employing institution.

TABLE 1-3   STRATEGIES FOR FISCALLY ACCOUNTABLE NURSING PRACTICE

1. Understand different reimbursement systems and what is covered under standard insurance systems.
2. Assess the resources the patient has available for heath care.
3. Be willing to discuss the cost of care with patients, families, and physicians.
4. Know what resources are available in the institution to assist patients and families with the costs of care.
5. Allocate professional nursing time appropriately, considering delegation to less-trained staff.
6. Use resources, supplies, and equipment to the maximum benefit of the patient. Question seemingly wasteful policies.
7. Charge out supplies accurately according to the institution's procedures.
8. Allocate your time based on patients' assessed needs.
9. Contribute to quality improvement initiatives by using data to produce improved clinical and fiscal outcomes.
10. Learn to speak "financial" so that you are able to communicate with decision makers and advocate for patients.

CHAPTER 2

Assessment

Assessment (data collection) is both the initial step in the nursing process and an ongoing component in every other step in the process. It is a systematic, deliberate process by which the nurse collects and analyzes data about the patient. Assessment is part of each activity the nurse does for and with the patient. The initial nursing assessment is the basis of the patient care plan, and later assessments contribute to revisions of and updates in the plan as the patient's condition changes. All individuals consistently use their five senses to assess changes in their environment and make the changes needed to adapt to it. One person may note the cold temperature and dress more warmly, while a second person is aware of a toothache and seeks dental care. Nurses also constantly seek information about the patient through their five senses and process it to identify changes in status and intervene appropriately.

Assessment is both the most basic and the most complex nursing skill. At the fundamental level, it is a beginning point for all nursing intervention. Without an assessment, the nurse has no idea how to begin helping a patient. At the most advanced level, assessment is a skill that distinguishes an expert nurse. An expert nurse can reliably say, "The patient just didn't look right" and often can predict significant changes in patients' conditions. Assessment is a complex and high level skill that must be practiced to achieve excellence. It is infinitely more complex than changing a sterile dressing or inserting an intravenous (IV) line.

Assessing (Data Collection)	=	Observation of Patient	+	Interview of Patient, Family, Other Nurses	+	Exam- ination of Patient	+	Medical Record Review

DATA COLLECTION

Initially, a nursing student collects data on an individual patient, but families, groups, and communities can all be the focus of a nursing assessment by more advanced nurses. While the student may focus on an individual patient initially, it is essential that the student recognize the uniqueness of the patient's culture. Often nurses complete their assessment from the perspective of their own culture, with little consideration of the patient's culture. What is considered "normal" in one culture may be unacceptable in another. As students become more experienced with assessment, family relationships and support systems, food preferences, communication styles, and health care beliefs are all included as aspects of patient assessment. Near the end of each chapter there is a section with the heading "Culturally Competent Nursing Care." That section will help a beginning nursing student develop an awareness of the cultural uniqueness of patients.

Because human beings are extraordinarily complex and because assessment is an ongoing process, there is the potential for nurses to collect an overwhelming amount of data. It is unrealistic to think that a nurse will record every bit of information that can be obtained. One component of the skill of assessment is the ability of the nurse to collect only *relevant* data. The nursing care plan is only as good as the data that go into it. A saying used by data analysts nicely illustrates this point: "Garbage in, garbage out."

Data Collection Format

Beginning nursing students often are required to complete patient data collection assignments. Often these assignments are very lengthy and time-consuming. The purpose of such an assignment is to assist the student in doing a comprehensive data review and avoid errors of omission. After the student has demonstrated proficiency in this skill, an abbreviated data collection format similar to the one used by staff nurses is recommended. Several examples of such forms will be used throughout this book.

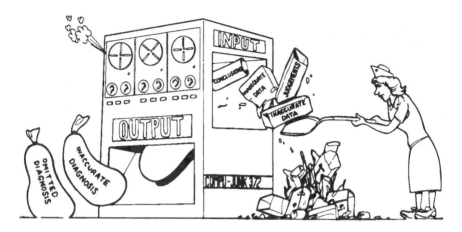

FIGURE 2-1.   Garbage in, garbage out.

Most hospitals and other health care institutions use a form to guide the collection of data when the nurse is admitting the patient. This form is usually labeled *Nursing Admission Assessment.* The structure of this form varies with the institution. A structured form is used to avoid omitting data in important human response areas and to give the patient an opportunity to discuss problems or request information in these areas. For example, when nurses (students and staff) complete an admission assessment, they frequently avoid initiating any discussion of sexuality or sexual behavior either by skipping the item completely or by marking the item "NA," which means "not applicable." Although this may enhance the student's comfort level at the time, it does not contribute to a comprehensive assessment of the patient. The nursing admission form includes this category, thus identifying it as important and encouraging nurses to do a more complete assessment even though there may initially be hesitancy or discomfort in asking questions in this area.

MASLOW'S BASIC NEED FRAMEWORK.   One assessment framework that is frequently used to guide the collection of data is based on the work of the psychologist Abraham Maslow (1968), who postulated that all human beings have common basic needs that can be arranged in a hierarchical order (Table 2-1). Maslow further theorized that basic physical needs must be met to some degree before higher level needs can be met.

Basic physical needs such as food, fluid, and oxygen are considered survival needs and must be met, or at least partially met, if life is to continue. They are the lowest level of needs and are usually partially satisfied before higher level needs are satisfied. The nursing care of critically ill patients usually focuses on physiological needs and safety needs to prevent physical harm. When the patient improves and life is no longer threatened, the satisfaction of higher level needs gains in importance. Higher level needs begin with security needs and continue through self-actualization needs.

TABLE 2-1   COMMON BASIC HUMAN NEEDS

1. Physiological needs—needs that must be met, or at least partially met, for survival
2. Safety and security needs—things that make a person feel safe and comfortable
3. Love and belonging needs—the need to give and receive love and affection
4. Esteem needs—things that make people feel good about themselves; pride in abilities and accomplishments
5. Self-actualization needs—the need to continue to grow and change; working toward future goals

Using Maslow's theory of basic needs, consider the following data and their relationship to basic needs:

1.   PHYSIOLOGICAL NEEDS
—temperature 103° F
—respiration 36 per minute
—liquid stool four times in 1 hour
—complains of sharp continuous pain in right lower quadrant

2.   SAFETY/SECURITY NEED
—sleeps with night-light
—"You won't forget me down in x-ray, will you?"
—"Last time I was in the hospital, I got my roommate's pill by accident."

3.   LOVE AND BELONGING
—parents are with Billy (hospitalized child)
—"We were married 40 years when my wife died. I miss her so much."

4.   SELF-ESTEEM
—"I can't even control my bowels—just like a baby."
—"I can't go to physical therapy without a shower and a shave."

5.   SELF-ACTUALIZATION
—"My children are grown with families of their own. Raising them has been my biggest accomplishment."
—"Teaching nursing students is more than a job. I feel like I'm contributing to their development and to the profession."
—"There is so much to learn about caring for my baby."

The data recorded within each category may indicate the current status of need satisfaction, alterations in meeting the need, or perhaps interferences in meeting the need. By collecting data in each of these need categories, the nurse develops a format for systematically considering the total patient rather than viewing an illness or a symptom. Comprehensive nursing care results from a

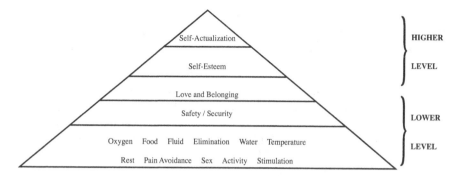

FIGURE 2-2. Maslow's hierarchy of human needs.

consideration of the total patient. At the end of this chapter there is an assessment form that uses Maslow's hierarchy of needs as an organizing framework.

HENDERSON'S COMPONENTS OF NURSING CARE.   Another framework that may be used to structure the nursing admission assessment was developed by the nurse-author Virginia Henderson. She described 14 needs or components of nursing care that a nurse may help the patient perform:

1. Breathe normally
2. Eat and drink adequately
3. Eliminate body waste
4. Move and maintain desirable posture
5. Sleep and rest
6. Select suitable clothing, dress and undress
7. Maintain body temperature
8. Keep the body clean and well groomed and protect the integument
9. Avoid dangers in the environment and avoid injuring others
10. Communicate with others
11. Worship according to one's faith
12. Work in such a way that there is a sense of accomplishment
13. Play, or participate in various forms of recreation
14. Learn, discover, or satisfy the curiosity that leads to "normal" development and health, and use available health facilities (Henderson, 1978)

After reading Henderson's list of nursing activities, the nurse can readily adapt the list to a data collection format. For example, the following questions and observations relate to Henderson's activities:

Activity 1. Breathe normally.   The nurse counts the respirations, observes the depth of breathing and the presence of retractions or nasal flaring, and uses a stethoscope to listen for lung sounds. The nurse may also ask the patient such questions as: Do you ever feel short of breath? What activity causes this? Do you

have any allergies that make you congested or that make it difficult to breathe? Do you ever experience nosebleeds? The nurse also examines the nailbeds and extremities for color, warmth, and capillary refill. All these observations indicate the level of oxygenation.

Activity 2. Eat and drink adequately. The nurse may ask the patient to describe a normal day's diet, when the major meal of the day is taken, and foods that cause the patient problems and to describe the resulting problems. The height, weight, and triceps skinfold may all be measured as a part of these data.

GORDON'S FUNCTIONAL HEALTH PATTERNS.   A third schema that is being used to structure nursing assessment is functional health pattern typology developed by Gordon (1982). Gordon proposes that the nurse assess the response pattern of the patient in 11 areas and then evaluate to determine if the pattern is functional or dysfunctional for a particular patient. The functional patterns specified by Gordon include

1. Health Perception–Health Management Pattern
2. Nutritional-Metabolic Pattern
3. Elimination Pattern
4. Activity-Exercise Pattern
5. Sleep-Rest Pattern
6. Cognitive-Perceptual Pattern
7. Self-Perception–Self-Concept Pattern
8. Role-Relationship Pattern
9. Sexuality-Reproductive Pattern
10. Coping–Stress Tolerance Pattern
11. Value-Belief Pattern

NANDA'S HUMAN RESPONSE PATTERNS.   Another structure that has implications for an assessment format is the proposal by the North American Nursing Diagnosis Association (NANDA). This is an international group that has provided leadership in an effort to develop nursing diagnoses. The purpose of this organization is to develop, refine, and promote a taxonomy of nursing diagnostic terminology of general use to professional nurses (NANDA Bylaws, Article 1, Section 2) (Carroll-Johnson, 1991). Taxonomy here refers to an orderly classification of nursing diagnoses. In 1998 at the 13th NANDA conference, the taxonomy committee proposed a new Taxonomy II to the membership. This taxonomy would classify nursing diagnoses on six axes (diagnostic concept, acuity, unit of care, developmental stage, potentiality, and descriptor) and 12 domains of health patterns (nutrition, elimination, cognition, etc.). This new taxonomy has not yet been approved, and nurses are encouraged to critically review the taxonomy and send feedback to the organization.

NURSING THEORIES.   The ultimate goal of nursing theory is to guide nursing practice. It is common for a school of nursing or a hospital to say that its nursing practice is based on a certain nursing theory.

An example of such a practice might be the application of Orem's self-care deficit theory (1985). This nursing theory states that the patient has health-related limitations in providing self-care. Thus, it is the role of the nurse to assist the patient in developing an optimal level of self-care. The nurse using this theory would focus on collecting data relative to self-care. For example, is the patient able to have an adequate nutritional intake; is the patient able to perform bowel and bladder elimination unassisted?

Another example of a nursing theory that could be used to guide assessment is the adaptation model of Sister Callista Roy. In this model, the human person is viewed as an adaptive system in constant interaction with its internal and external environment (Alligood and Tomey, 1997). The focus of nursing is to promote the adaptive behaviors of the patient. During the assessment phase the nurse would gather data related to the patient's responses in each of the four adaptive modes: physiology, self-concept, role function, and interdependence.

HUMAN GROWTH AND DEVELOPMENT.   Any format used for data collection is acceptable as long as it is thorough and comprehensive and considers both the physiological and psychosocial aspects of the human being. In addition, any data collection approach must also include consideration of the individual's level of growth and development. Each chronological age has corresponding developmental tasks, both physical and psychosocial. A developmental task may be thought of as a job, a hurdle, a challenge, or an accomplishment related to a particular chronological age span. Illness may interfere with the completion of developmental tasks appropriate to an age span or with progression to the next developmental level. During illness an individual may even regress to an earlier level of development. For example, a 3-year-old who has been toilet trained for 6 months may begin bed wetting again during hospitalization. An adolescent who has been menstruating for 6 months may cease to menstruate during a lengthy confinement in a body cast. Other individuals may appear to arrest at a developmental level during the stress of illness and hospitalization. For example, an infant may fail to begin to crawl and stand during illness. The infant may remain at the developmental level achieved before hospitalization and show very little new learning until the stress of hospitalization and illness is reduced.

Thus, it is important for nurses to include an assessment of the developmental levels and tasks associated with each stage so that they can recognize and understand variations from normal age-related development in patients. By recognizing that a child is regressing to an earlier level or is failing to keep up with peers' development, the nurse may be able to work with parents and other hospital staff to reduce the damaging influence that hospitalization is having on that child's development. A nurse who has a knowledge of developmental levels and the associated tasks will be able to further individualize nursing care. For example, adolescent developmental tasks focus on self-identity. While caring for adolescents, the nurse might choose a nonauthoritative approach that would give the teen the maximum amount of choice. Similarly, a school-aged child's developmental level focuses on independence and project completion. Nursing care that encourages the child's self-care will promote developmental growth. Table 2-2

TABLE 2-2   MAJOR DEVELOPMENTAL TASKS

1. Infant—1 month to year
    —developing a sense of trust and belonging from relationship with mother and father
    —differentiating self from environment
    —learning to eat solid foods, walk, explore, communicate
2. Toddler—1–3 years
    —developing will power, independence
    —learning to feed self, run, communicate verbally, control elimination
    —exploring environment
3. Preschool—3–6 years
    —developing sexual identity
    —developing sense of initiative
    —working on autonomy, dressing self, washing
    —developing sense of time, space, distance
    —developing imagination
    —playing cooperatively
4. School age—6 to puberty
    —developing a sense of work; planning and carrying out projects
    —learning the skills for survival in the child's culture
    —developing modesty
    —learning to read, calculate
    —developing neuromuscular coordination
    —learning to control emotions
5. Adolescent—12–20 years
    —developing physical maturity
    —developing autonomy from home and family
    —developing self-identity
    —coping with body image changes
    —identifying with peer group
6. Young adult—18–40 years
    —establishing enduring close physical and emotional relationships
    —childbearing, child rearing
    —establishing financial security
    —community responsibility
    —social interaction with peers
7. Middle adult—40–65 years of age
    —separating from children
    —establishing self in job
    —adapting to aged parents
    —adapting to physiological changes of aging
    —adjusting to altered relationship with spouse
8. Older adult
    —accepting own life as valuable and appropriate
    —adapting to reduced physical health and strength
    —adapting to possible death of spouse
    —adjusting to retirement income
    —developing relationships with new family members
    —adapting to change in living location and style

gives a brief summary of some of the major developmental tasks corresponding to chronological age.

Data Collection Skills

When a patient is admitted to the hospital, the nurse begins planning nursing care. This is done by using the skills of data collection. Observation, interview, examination, and medical record review are four methods the nurse uses to collect data. Although there are multiple sources the nurse may use for data collection, the patient is always the primary source. Even if the patient is unable to communicate verbally, the nurse can elicit valuable data by using observation and examination skills. Additional data sources may be the patient's past medical record (chart), significant others, and other persons giving care to the patient. Professional journals, reference texts, and clinical nurse specialists are also important sources of data.

Nursing observations result in objective data. *Objective data* are factual data that are observed by the nurse and could be noted by any other skilled observer. During the assessment phase of the nursing process, the nurse describes the signs or behaviors observed without drawing conclusions or making interpretations. At this point the nurse focuses on establishing a comprehensive data base about the patient. Premature interpretation and analysis based on incomplete data may lead to errors. See Table 2-3 for examples of objective data. The column of judgments and conclusions demonstrates the interpretations of one individual nurse. Consider that "neatly groomed" may mean different things to different individuals and different cultures, whereas "hair combed, makeup applied" is concise and descriptive.

TABLE 2-3   OBJECTIVE DATA

Objective Data	Judgments and Conclusions
Hair combed, makeup applied	Improved body image
Drags right leg when walking	Intoxicated
Tremors of both hands	Patient very afraid
250 cc dark amber urine	Voided large amount
Patient in bed, covers over head. facing wall; no verbal response to questions	Patient depressed
Administered own 8 A.M. insulin, using sterile technique	Understands self-administration of insulin
Ate cereal, juice, toast, coffee	Good appetite
Requests pain med q2h	Low pain tolerance

Contrasted with objective data are subjective data. *Subjective data* consist of information given verbally by the patient. Examples of this type of data are the following statements:

"I feel so nervous."
"My stomach is burning."
"I want to be alone now."

From the examples of subjective data listed above each nurse could infer many different interpretations. For example, the nurse might guess that the patient is nervous, fearing a diagnosis of cancer. This interpretation is not justified on the basis of the patient's statement. The patient could be nervous for many different reasons. The task during data collection is merely to observe, collect, and record data. Subjective data such as the examples in Table 2-4 are best recorded as direct quotes, thus providing the reader with the original information.

OBSERVATION.   Observation is a high level nursing skill that requires a great deal of practice. Consider a grocery shopping trip. Even though it is possible to have shopped at the store several times previously, few people can successfully recall all the items they need without a list or even find the location of all the items they wish to purchase. The skills of observation and recall are difficult, but like all other skills, they can be learned with systematic study and practice. An inexperienced student nurse will find it hard to perform nursing tasks and simultaneously continue the observation process, yet it is this ability to perform constant, ongoing observation that is essential to assessment. For example, nursing students giving a first bedbath are concentrating so hard on the task that they may be unable to make observations or converse with the patient. As students gain skill in giving physical care, they can shift their attention to the total patient and begin to collect data through observation. They are now able to observe the skin condition, color, and temperature while bathing a patient. The quality, depth, and effort of respirations can be noted. The ability of the patient to move, as well as any pain associated with movement, is noted. While giving a back rub, the skilled student can view the skin over the lower back, which is often an area of breakdown. The condition of the mucous membrane is noted during oral

TABLE 2-4   SUBJECTIVE DATA

Subjective Data	Judgments and Conclusions
"Get out of my room."	Patient is hostile
"I know something is wrong with my baby.	Patient is anxious
"This catheter is killing me."	Patient has pain
"Where am I? How did I get here?"	Patient is confused
"I'm afraid they will find cancer when they operate."	Patient is worried about surgery

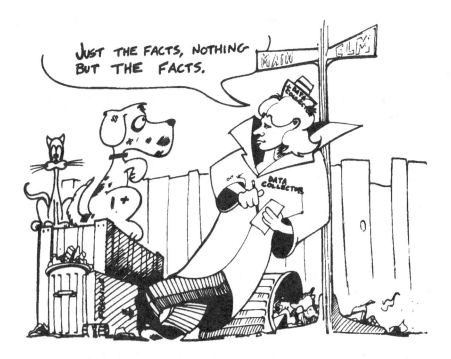

FIGURE 2-3.   The nurse records observations without drawing conclusions.

hygiene. The ability of the patient to tolerate activity also may be observed as the nurse watches for signs of fatigue during and after the bath.

INTERVIEW.   The interview is a structured form of communication that the nurse uses to collect data. Both the ability to ask questions and the ability to listen are essential to successful interviews.

The nursing history or nursing admission assessment is one type of interview. This is completed by the nurse at the time of admission. The focus of the nursing history is the patient's response to actual or potential health problems. As a part of this process, the nurse reviews the patient's past health history and coping methods that have been effective or ineffective. Data related to the patient's life-style may also help identify health risk factors. The nursing history is not a duplicate of the medical history, which has the disease process as its main focus. The purpose of the nursing history is to enable the nurse to plan nursing care for the patient. The nurse clearly and directly conveys this purpose to the patient at the beginning of the interview. The nurse may say something like the following:

> "Mr. Jones, I am Ms. Murray. I am the registered nurse who will be responsible for planning the nursing care you will receive while you are here. I would like to spend about a half hour with you now talking about your health history and completing this nursing admission form. This information will help me work with you to begin to plan your nursing care."

Observation is a high-level nursing skill . . .

"What you want are facts, not opinions—for who can have any opinion of any value as to whether the patient is better or worse, excepting the constant medical attendant, or the really observing nurse? The most important practical lesson that can be given to nurses is to teach them what to observe—how to observe—what symptoms indicate improvement—what the reverse—which are of importance—which are of none—which are the evidence of neglect—and what kind of neglect."   *p. 105*

"But if you cannot get the habit of observation one way or other, you had better give up the being a nurse, for it is not your calling, however kind and anxious you may be."   *p. 113*

"In dwelling upon the importance of sound observation, it must never be lost sight of what observation is for. It is not for the sake of piling up miscellaneous information or curious facts, but for the sake of saving life and increasing health and comfort."   *p. 125*

Florence Nightingale, *Notes on Nursing: What It Is and What It Is Not.* From an unabridged republication of the first American edition as published in 1860. (1969) New York: Dover Publications.

Note that the nurse has introduced herself in a professional manner and has clearly stated her professional accountability. If the institution uses them, this would be the appropriate time for the nurse to give the patient a business card that also indicates a hospital telephone number where messages may be left when the nurse is not on the unit. This introduction is in contrast to "Hi, I'm Anne and I'm your nurse. I need to ask you some questions."

Before beginning the nursing history, the nurse helps make the patient as comfortable as possible. This would include assessing for pain and doing what is necessary to reduce discomfort. It may also be helpful to offer the patient the opportunity to go to the bathroom before beginning. Note that the nurse in the above example also gave the patient some indication of the amount of time the interview would take. This is helpful to a patient who may be expecting visitors or perhaps planning to make a telephone call. The nurse may also offer the patient a beverage if that is medically permitted. This may help put the patient at ease and contribute to openness in the interview process. It is also helpful if the nurse sits during the interview at a level where eye contact between the nurse and the patient can be easily maintained. This reduces the superior (nurse standing)–inferior (patient in bed) feeling of the nurse–patient relationship and conveys that the nurse has time to listen.

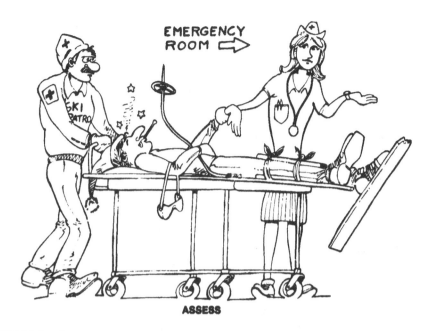

EMERGENCY
ROOM ⇨

ASSESS

FIGURE 2-4.   The nurse collects data through interviewing, observations, examinations, and chart review.

Most hospitals have a nursing history form that the nurse fills out on admission. This form guides or structures the interview, but the form is only a starting point. The nurse uses professional judgment to clarify areas of confusion or elicit additional relevant data. The nurse does not form judgments or conclusions during the data collection phase or rely on the judgments or conclusions of the patient. For example, the nurse does not ask the patient, "Do you have problems with your bowel movements?" To this question the patient may easily reply no. This illustrates a judgment made by the patient. Contrast this with the following dialogue between a nurse and a patient:

NURSE: What is your normal pattern of bowel movements (BM)?
PATIENT: I have a BM about every other day.
NURSE: Has this changed since you broke your hip?
PATIENT: Yes—I feel constipated almost all the time.
NURSE: Have you done anything to treat your constipation?
PATIENT: Yes—I started to take a laxative both in the morning and in the evening. Sometimes it works too much and I get diarrhea, and other times I still feel constipated.

In this case the nurse has asked a series of open-ended questions (questions that cannot be answered yes or no) to assess the patient's health pattern and elicit a more comprehensive picture of the health pattern. The beginning nurse may

wish to use the following series of questions to guide the assessment of each health area (Table 2-5):

1. What is your normal pattern (or behavior)?
2. Has your current health problem (illness, injury) affected your normal pattern (or behavior)?
3. Have you done anything to help maintain or restore patterns (behavior) affected by your current health problem?

The nurse probably will find it helpful to take notes and actually complete most of the form during the interview process. Some explanation is always given to the patient. The nurse may say, "Mr. Jones, I will be taking notes as we talk to make sure that I am accurate in recording this information." At the end of the interview it is helpful if the nurse summarizes the notes for the patient, especially those areas where the current health problem has affected function or behavior. This contributes to the sense of trust in the nurse–patient relationship and gives the patient the opportunity to add or correct data.

Frequently, beginning nursing students are uncomfortable eliciting a nursing history. Students often state that they feel they are prying into personal matters. Students may be reassured that the patient has the right to refuse to discuss any topic and that this right must be respected. When patients do choose to reveal personal data, nurses and students are responsible for assuring that the shared information remains confidential. Such data will remain within the context of the professional relationship and will be shared only with those who need the information to provide care.

The formal nursing interview is not primarily intended to be a treatment in and of itself but is an organized format for data collection. Frequently, however, the patient has a need to express feelings or share things that are worrisome, and the nursing interview provides the opportunity and the uninterrupted attention of the nurse.

TABLE 2-5   OPEN-ENDED QUESTIONS TO GUIDE ASSESSMENT OF HEALTH PATTERNS

Focus	Nurse	Patient Example
1. Normal pattern	"What do you usually eat for breakfast?"	"I like eggs and toast with lots of butter."
2. Effect of medical problems	"Has this changed since you've had this problem?"	"Yes, I really get heartburn from this."
3. Coping strategies	"Have you done anything different to help this?"	"Well, mostly I just skip breakfast or eat plain cereal. That helps."

Often therapeutic communication may be the most appropriate skill to offer the patient . . .

I remember it as if it were yesterday—and it happened over 20 years ago! I was a third-year student nurse in a diploma program, and I was working 3–11:30 P.M. on a rehabilitation unit. Most patients on this unit had survived a major trauma and were transferred to the unit for rehabilitation. Most of the patients were paraplegic or quadriplegic with little hope of return of function.

On this particular evening I had completed most of my work settling patients for the night. One young man, John, was very restless. He had been injured in a manufacturing accident and was permanently paralyzed from the waist down. He was very handsome, intelligent, and recently married at age 26 years. I had given him a muscle relaxant and a back rub and assisted with hygiene. Though he usually retired early and slept soundly, tonight he seemed troubled and moody, not his usual self. At 11:10 I walked past his room and noticing his light still on, I entered his room to find him staring at the ceiling. "How's it going, John?" I asked as I settled into a chair at his bedside. "Do you want some company?" He invited me to stay and admitted he was at "rock bottom." We talked a long time, and in the conversation that followed he revealed that he and his wife had always wanted children and that there was still the chance that physically he could father a child. "But," he confided, "what would a kid think of having a father in a wheelchair?"

I told him! For my father had multiple sclerosis and had suffered a progressively degenerative course to where he was ultimately a quadriplegic. I told him of the tough times, of the things I missed or envied in my friends' fathers, but I told him too of the love and support of my father . . . of the closeness of our relationship . . . of my respect for and pride in my father. "But," John said, "that was because you were a girl. What if I had a son?" I couldn't answer for my brother, I said, but I could describe my family life. After a long time, John said, "Thank you, you've helped." I finished my charting and when I left the unit, his light was out and he was sleeping.

The informal aspect of the nursing interview is the conversation between the nurse and the patient in the course of giving nursing care. The close relationship often developed while the nurse is giving physical care frequently enables the patient to express concerns. A nurse who can skillfully give physical care is then free to simultaneously focus attention on what the patient is saying.

The planned, deliberate communication the nurse uses to help identify and meet the health care needs of the patient is called *therapeutic communication*. Like other nursing skills, therapeutic communication requires practice to be

effective. It may be difficult for beginning nursing students to give physical care while simultaneously engaging in therapeutic communication. Often, for example, the nurse uses the time spent giving a bedbath as an opportunity for therapeutic communication. This is often an unhurried, private time for conversation between the nurse and the patient. With practice, the nurse is able to focus on what the patient is saying. During this communication the nurse also continues to make observations.

At other times, the nurse will plan a period of time for the sole purpose of engaging in therapeutic communication. This too may be difficult for a beginning student who may feel uncomfortable approaching patients without a technical task (such as taking a blood pressure) to "do for" the patient. Often therapeutic communications may be the most appropriate skill to offer the patient. This may be the case when a patient is afraid or discouraged or has just been told of a serious diagnosis.

EXAMINATION.   The third activity in data collection is examination. A complete physical examination is a skill beyond the scope of most registered nurses and usually is done by nurses with advanced education and training. A partial physical examination that is limited to an area of practice or that focuses on a specific problem is a skill expected of all nurses. Before beginning the physical process of examination, the nurse establishes a relationship with the patient. The nurse always precedes the examination with an explanation of the procedure and requests the patient's permission to proceed. The nurse provides for the patient's privacy, closing doors and pulling curtains as necessary. The nurse checks with patients and asks if the would prefer if their visitors wait outside the room before beginning. The nurse might say something like, "Mrs. Jones, I'd like to do a physical examination now with your permission. If you feel any discomfort, will you please tell me? I'll begin by checking your eyes and ears." When doing only a partial physical examination, the nurse might state, "I'd like to take a look at your stitches and the drain site to make sure everything is healing."

The nurse is then ready to begin a physical examination of the patient. The nurse may choose to conduct a total body assessment or to focus on one or more specific areas, such as lung sounds, stitches, or a wound or a drain. If a patient complains of generalized pain, the nurse may conduct a very thorough examination. In contrast, if a child in the emergency room fell from a bicycle and shows the nurse a large bleeding laceration on the elbow, this might be the initial focus of the examination. It is important that the nurse conduct a thorough examination as soon as possible, since internal injuries that are not so readily apparent may be present.

In obtaining this examination data, the nurse uses a systematic approach to avoid omissions. For nursing students, the particular curriculum of a school may require a certain approach. Hospitals may, by the forms they provide, structure the examination done by a practicing nurse. It really does not matter which approach is used as long as it is methodical and the nurse uses it consistently to

gain a high degree of skill. One nurse may follow a *cephalocaudal* (head-to-toe) approach, which begins with an assessment of the hair, skull, eyes, ears, nose, mouth, and facial skin and moves in a downward direction. Another nurse may select a *body system* approach, which may begin with a consideration of the respiratory system, moving to the digestive system, then to the cardiovascular system, and so forth. Any methodical, thorough approach is acceptable as long as it meets the need to gather relevant data that help identify health problems requiring nursing intervention.

During physical examination, the nurse uses senses and skills to gather information about the patient. *Visualization* is inspection of the patient's body. This is coupled with the use of the senses such as hearing, smelling (certain disease processes or physical changes are associated with characteristic odors), and touching. Visualization is often the most appropriate starting place for a physical examination because the nurse will not cause the patient any discomfort. The nurse also uses the skill of *auscultation*, which includes listening with a stethoscope to heart, lung, and bowel sounds. Next the nurse may palpate, or feel, the body. This may give the nurse information about organ position, body temperature, abnormal growths, abdominal rigidity, or the location of pain. Some nurses may be skilled in the use of *percussion*, the tapping of a body surface, usually with the fingers. This is done to elicit responses, usually in the form of sound or movement, that give information about an underlying body part. For example, it is common practice to percuss a distended abdomen for a drumlike sound indicating retained flatus (gas) in the bowel after abdominal surgery.

While it is necessary to establish a relationship with a patient before an examination, the examination itself can be a tool for showing concern and enhancing the relationship. It is the standard of care in most settings that the nurse take *five vital signs*: temperature (TPR), blood pressure (BP), and pain. The first four vital signs have been well integrated into nursing practice. There are customary protocols that direct how often nurses must take TPR and BP after surgery and before and after most procedures. The best clinical practice also dictates that each time nurses complete the assessment of TPR and BP, they also assess the patient for pain. It is a standard clinical practice to use a pain rating scale. The nurse asks the patient, "On a scale of zero to ten, if zero is no pain at all and ten is the worst pain imaginable, how would you rate your pain?" The nurse records this rating as the fifth vital sign. No recording of vital signs is complete without all five components. In addition to asking about pain, the nurse observes the patient for signs of pain. Some patients may be reluctant to tell the nurse for fear of being labeled a "wimp" or a "sissy." Other patients may attempt to be stoic and endure unnecessary pain, as that might be their idea of a "good patient." The nurse observes for less obvious signs of pain: Does the patient recoil when touched during physical examination or limp when walking? Are there facial signs that might indicate pain? All these signs are noted and recorded as the fifth vital sign. To take only four vital signs is a serious omission and creates a gap in clinical care. The nurse demonstrates concern for the patient by tak-

ing the patient's experience of pain seriously, assessing and recording it carefully, and intervening aggressively.

MEDICAL RECORD REVIEW.   The final activity in data collection is medical record review. The nurse reads a medical record (patient chart) to add to the comprehensive assessment. There are several purposes for reading the record:

- To guide the other activities of data collection based on high frequency health problems associated with medical diagnoses and treatments identified in the chart
- To relate the past health care history of the patient to the present episode
- To identify what medication the patient is taking so that the assessment can include the effectiveness of the medication and the occurrence of any side effects
- To understand interdisciplinary care planning, since each discipline evaluates the patient and records its conclusions and recommendations in the chart
- To understand the nursing diagnoses and interventions in past episodes in order to build on them
- To determine the presence and content of advance directives, that is, patients' written wishes regarding the extent and continuation of medical treatment in the event that they are unable to speak for themselves
- To understand other health team members' evaluations of the patient's clinical progress
- To clarify information found on the patient's Kardex or medication administration record

Beginning nursing students may find it more comfortable to read the chart and gather information from this source first. Some nursing faculty members discourage students from reading the chart until after they have interviewed the patient. This is done in an effort to stress to students that the patient and family are the most valuable sources of information. However, any assessment that does not include record review is incomplete. It is also important to understand that nursing is one component of the interdisciplinary patient care team. Many other disciplines are also essential in assuring that patients' needs are met. As nurses we collaborate with colleagues in other disciplines, and one way we communicate with them is through the patient record.

During the assessment phase the nurse has the potential to collect volumes of data about a patient. Throughout the process it is important to consider the significance of the data to the task at hand, which is identifying problems and planning nursing intervention. As the student practices data collection, skill is gained in eliciting and recording relevant data. It is also essential that the student learn to report data in a timely manner to the appropriate person. If the physician sees the patient once a day, and a major change in the patient's condition is noted after that visit, it is the responsibility of the nurse to report this immediately in addition to completing the necessary documentation.

CRITICAL THINKING FOR ASSESSMENT

The activities involved in the assessment phase of the nursing process involve critical thinking. All of a patient's care is based on an assessment that shows the nurse both the objective data and the patient's perception of the situation, at this time, at this stage of health, illness, or recovery. One of the best ways to provide care that meets the needs of the patient is to have an accurate and complete assessment that also focuses on important patient cues. Making judgments or decisions based on incomplete information is easy to do and is a common mistake of novice nurses and students in nursing. Make sure all your information is factual, whether you collected it yourself or someone else did. Be skeptical of abnormal or unusual findings and recheck them if you want to be a critical thinker.

Learn more about disease conditions and people's responses to illness and treatment to be more aware of clusters of data that indicate problems. Then, when your patient exhibits one of those data pieces, look for the other data in that cluster during your assessment. Put the data package together by clustering the data.

An elderly woman is not drinking fluids, and because of this, her IV must remain infusing. Yet she seems alert and capable of drinking. The critically thinking nurse identifies this minimal fluid intake as abnormal in an alert patient and then relates this to knowledge of culturally appropriate liquids and the temperatures of those liquids. The nurse looks for more related data to rule in or rule out this possible cause for the problem. The nurse discovers that the elderly woman will drink only hot fluids and the staff keeps bringing her ice water and cold beverages on her tray. To ask for hot fluids from the nurse would be disrespectful, and so the patient has said nothing. The nurse explains the need for the woman to drink fluid, which she begins to do immediately when she is brought hot water in her water pitcher.

A patient has an elevated temperature as reported by the nursing assistant. The critically thinking nurse goes in, rechecks the data, considers possible causes for this cue, and seeks out related data. Did the patient just drink something hot? Was the thermometer accurate? Are there any signs and symptoms of infection? How does the patient feel? What was the previous temperature? The nurse does not just call the physician and say, "The patient has a fever. What should we do?" The critically thinking nurse calls the doctor with the data clustered: "Rechecked temperature was 101 degrees; it was 99.8 four hours ago. The incision looks red about 2 inches out from the suture line, and the patient is complaining of chills and feels 'awful.' No antibiotics were ordered postoperatively."

Experienced nurses collect more pertinent cues from the patient than novice nurses do. As novice nurses (nursing students), you may not have enough knowledge to know the difference between important and unimportant patient cues, but you will learn. Expert nurses who use critical thinking during

assessment are more aware of common problems all patients may experience related to certain medical diagnoses, treatments, or surgery and focus assessment on ruling them in and out. You will learn this as your knowledge and experience increase over the course of your nursing program and clinical practice. Listed below are some questions to ask yourself as you assess your patients to stimulate critical thinking. Following that are two practice exercises to help you practice asking assessment questions and clustering data to reach a clinical judgment.

Prompts for Critical Thinking during Assessment

- What specific data do I need to collect based on the medical diagnosis, treatments, chief complaint, and chronic condition?
- What risk factors from the history may indicate a potential problem (nursing diagnosis) that can be prevented before it occurs?
- What are the high frequency problems (nursing diagnoses) for patients in this age group with this health problem/treatment, and did I seek out the presence of signs and symptoms indicating their development or occurrence?
- Did I get enough data focused on each potential problem to diagnose accurately?
- Did I use enough sources? What other data are needed?
- Did I recheck any abnormal or unexpected data to make sure those data were accurate?
- Did I follow up on patient cues, seeking out more data related to cues that might indicate a problem?
- Did I consider several causes for a sign or symptom and collect data associated with those causes?
- Did I see and hear what really was occurring or what I wanted to occur or what usually occurs? What assumptions or biases do I have in this situation?
- Did the patient's words match the behavior I observed? If not, did I clarify the discrepancy with the patient?
- Did I collect data on how age, sex, culture, and family might affect the meaning of illness, treatment, and recovery?
- What does the patient think? Does it differ from what the family, the doctor, or the nurses think?

CRITICAL THINKING PRACTICE EXERCISES DURING ASSESSMENT

What to Do with the IV?

It is 3 P.M., and you are getting the report for your 3–11:30 shift. Your patient is 1 day postop from a rotator cuff (shoulder) repair done late yesterday afternoon. He is 46 years old, has no history of medical problems, and has an IV of D5LR running at 125/hr. His physician's order for the IV fluids reads:

D5LR at 125 ml/hr; D/C IV when tolerating PO fluids
Ancef 1 g IVPB q6h × 3 doses

After reading the report, you go into this patient's room and find there are only 50 cc of IV fluid left in the IV bag. You need to decide what to do. Your choices are listed below:

1. Hang another bag of the D5LR.
2. Slow the IV down to a TVO (TKO) rate for the next hour or so; then either hang another bag of D5LR or discontinue the IV based on a new assessment.
3. Saline lock the IV (at your hospital this is a nursing decision).
4. Discontinue the IV by removing the needle.

What additional data will you need to obtain from the patient or the chart to make this decision? Write out your specific assessment questions below or on a separate piece of paper. (Be specific with your question. Do not ask for a judgment; ask for the data.) Look below to see what areas are important to assess and what specific data you need to obtain to make the correct decision. The data from each scenario will result in a different IV choice based on the patient's current postoperative status.

DATA KEY TO IV PROBLEM

Data nurse should ask for	Scenario A	Scenario B	Scenario C
Food/fluids taken			
Nausea?	Yes	Early A.M.; OK now	No
Vomiting?	Yes; X2	Last night; not today	No
How much fluid taken?	Ice chips/sips	11–7 A.M. = 100 ml	11–7 A.M. = 350 ml
I&O?		7–3 P.M. = 250 ml	7–3 P.M. = 850 ml
Medications			
No. doses of Ancef given	3 doses given	2 doses given; last dose due at 4 P.M.	3 doses given
Wound			
Site inspection	No S&S of problem	No S&S of problem	No S&S of problem
Bowel/elimination			
Bowel sounds?	Faint upper 2 quad	Good all 4 quad	Good all 4 quad

(continued on next page)

DATA KEY TO IV PROBLEM (Continued)

Data nurse should ask for	Scenario A	Scenario B	Scenario C
Passing gas?	No	Just now	Yes
Abdominal distension?	Slight	No	No
Urinary/elimination Urine output	7–3 P.M. = 400 ml	7–3 P.M. = 600 ml	7–3 P.M. = 750 ml
Vital signs	101–96–17	98–82–16	97.6–78–15
Pain	Rated as 6	Rated as 4	Rated as 3

Answers with Rationale:

1. Assessment questions from each of the data clusters above is the goal.
2. Solution and Rationale

Scenario A
"Hang another bag" is the correct action; N&V, unable to meet own hydration needs (needs at least 100–150 ml/hr of oral intake for several hours to show that at that rate patient could reach normal daily intake of 1500 ml); not passing gas; faint bowel sounds means minimal peristalsis and food would stay in stomach, possibly causing more nausea or more abdominal distension; urine output still low (some dehydration?), not ready to force fluids to increase oral intake because still nauseated; IV not needed for Ancef since all doses given, but because patient is running a temperature, doctor may order more IV doses.

Scenario B
Saline lock or slow down; needs last dose of Ancef at 4 P.M.; IV site is okay; will encourage oral intake over next 1–2 hrs to see if he can take several hundred ml without any nausea; plan to discontinue the IV after last Ancef dose if oral intake good and no problems.

Scenario C
Discontinue IV; excellent I&O; no N&V; good BS and passing gas; no abnormal VS; all antibiotics given.

What's for Supper?

Mrs. Anderson had emergency surgery for her fractured leg at 5:10 A.M. Her postoperative orders include the following:

**Clear liquids postnausea, advance as tolerated
D5LR at 125/hr; D/C IV when tolerating fluids
Ampicillin 1 g IV q6h × 4 doses**

She has an IV of D5LR running at 125 cc/hr. You are her 3–11 P.M. nurse and are just coming out of report. You need to order her a supper tray. Your clinical reasoning problem is to collect enough data to make a decision on which type of diet to order for her supper tray:

_____ clear liquids or no tray at all; ice chips

_____ full liquids

_____ regular diet

Based on this minimal information, what additional data would you obtain from the patient or from the chart? Write out your specific assessment questions below (do not ask for a judgment or decision). Look below to see what areas are important to assess and what specific data to obtain to make the correct decision. The data from each scenario will result in a different diet choice based on the patient's current postoperative status.

DATA KEY TO DIET PROBLEM

Data nurse should ask for	Scenario A	Scenario B
Fluid/food intake and response		
Nausea?	Yes	No
Vomiting?	Yes; just gave compazine	No
Feeling hungry?	No	Yes
What amount of fluids has she taken so far?	1/2 cup	cl liquid lunch 400 ml
What type of fluids?	Ice chips	Crackers at 2 P.M.
Elimination/bowel/peristalsis		
Abdominal distension?	Some	No
Bowel sounds present? All 4 quadrants?	Faint, upper quadrant only	Very active all 4
Passing gas?	No	Yes
Type of anesthesia	General	Epidural

Answers with Rationale:

1. Assessment questions from each of the data clusters above is the goal.
2. Solution and Rationale

Scenario A
Potential or actual problem: not tolerating fluids; not ready for diet to be advanced; "no tray or clear liquids" is the correct diet to order; she is not tolerating even ice chips at this point; still having N&V; advancing diet probably would make her S&S worse; bowel hypoactive; foods/fluids entering stomach will not advance normally.

Full liquid diet is not as good a choice based on lack of tolerance of clear liquids but is not as inappropriate as a regular diet.
Regular diet is an inappropriate choice based on physical data.

Scenario B
Data indicate absence of any problems; tolerating fluids; ready to advance diet; "regular diet" is the best choice; bowel sounds active; passing gas and tolerating clear fluids and crackers without N&V indicate a readiness for more solid foods; epidural anesthesia affects bowel functioning minimally compared with general anesthesia, and the surgery did not involve the abdomen, which might have reduced perisitalsis and caused more postoperative GI problems.

Full liquids is not a wrong choice, but the data indicate you could advance the diet more aggressively, but at least the diet was advanced.

Clear liquids show no advancement in diet order when all data indicate that advancement is appropriate.

CULTURALLY COMPETENT CARE DURING ASSESSMENT

As a nurse, your assessments of your patients will include cultural aspects. Sometimes, though, because we view others through our own ethnocentrism, we assume or fail to assess because we do not understand the impact of an individual's culture on health and health care. Western medicine's values and treatments may be frightening to someone from another culture and conflict with traditional forms of healing. How can we know? We *assess* and do not *assume*. We ask and we listen. Learn more about cultures, starting with your own. Know generalizations about the cultures you work with, but do not stereotype patients. "Some women I have worked with who have come from China want to drink only a special healing tea they bring from home after giving birth. Is this something you had planned to do, or are there some fluids I can get you here that you would prefer?" Assessing is the key rather than saying, "Since you are from China, you must want to drink only that special tea you make from herbs." That would be stereotyping.

Assessment requires communication, but this is often difficult when the nurse and the patient do not speak the same language. Determine the patient's ability to understand and respond in English. If this is a problem, get a professional interpreter before beginning an assessment. Get an interpreter who is not a family member or a friend to allow for patient privacy, confidentiality, and accurate communication of medical terms. For example, one family was using its 12-year-old son as an interpreter, and the doctor was talking about a magnetic resonance image (MRI), a type of x-ray, to help make the diagnosis. The son, not knowing medical terms, used "microwave" in the translation. Health care facilities frequently have lists of interpreters available. Do not just speak more loudly and slowly, which is our natural tendency when we are not being understood. Provide translated assessment questions that the patient and family can respond to for the interpreter. When using an interpreter, talk to the patient, not to the interpreter. Do not use slang, technical language, abbreviations, or long sentences. If language is a problem, use nonverbal aids such as the faces pain assessment scale rather than a number rating or descriptive scale.

Do not use the patient's first name initially; titles may be expected, and using the first name may be viewed as disrespectful. Ask how the patient prefers to be addressed. Patients may address you as "Nurse" rather than using your name; this is a sign of respect.

Take nonverbal cues from the family. As the nurse, if you talk to the patient and the patient turns to another family member, who then responds for the patient, you might ask whether questions should be directed to that person. In some cultures, the elder male or female is the appropriate family member to address. This person makes health care decisions, not the patient. Remember, continued eye contact from the patient to you may be inappropriate in his or her culture. Lack of eye contact may not be a sign of inattention.

Prompts for Culturally Competent Nursing Care during Assessment

- Are you able to understand and speak English fairly well? Is it your native language?
- What do you think caused your problem?
- Is there anything that might have prevented this problem?
- How long have you been having this problem? (Remember that some cultures have a less defined sense of time, and so "long time" and "short time" will need clarifying in terms of other life events as time markers.)
- What have you done so far to try to get better?
- Have you been using any medications, herbs, or other treatments?
- What kind of treatments or medicine do you (your family) think you should receive here?
- Will someone from your family be staying with you most of the time?
- Are there any special clothing or dressing preferences that you want to continue while you are here?

- Are there any daily religious needs that you want to continue while you are here?
- Do you have any special food preferences that you think will help you? Any foods or fluids you should not have or that make you sick?
- Do you prefer hot or cold liquids in the pitcher at your bedside?
- Are there any questions you or your family would like to ask me or the doctor?
- How would you like to be addressed?

ASSESSMENT

The Circle of Life

The collection of pertinent data during the patient assessment is the most critical aspect of the nursing process. A good assessment was never as important as it was the day I assisted five Hindu students in the emergency room. The five college students had just arrived from India and were looking forward to celebrating their first Fourth of July. However, an unplanned detour into our emergency room brought the five students in after an unthinkable accident. The group had driven its car into a telephone pole not far from the hospital. Three of the young men were critically injured. The other two, a man and a young woman, were both in fair condition and were able to assist the hospital staff with the identification of the students who could not speak for themselves. As I was the nursing supervisor on duty, it became my responsibility to assess the situation, assist with the placement of the students into the hospital's ICU, and coordinate the efforts for the one student who was not to survive the ordeal.

I quickly gained much-needed information on the customs and beliefs of the Hindu religion. Five calls to India were made that evening from our emergency room. Five explanations of the medical conditions, treatment options, and future plans were communicated. Five regrets for this unfortunate incident were made to family members who would have given anything to be with their children at a time when family should have been the most important thing. The poise, grace, and respect that these young people exhibited in the face of tragedy were inspiring. The two students who were able to participate wanted the death of their companion to be as traditional as possible. The death needed to be comfortable and peaceful. The death needed to be a spiritual experience that could allow the young man's sole to transfer to its next existence.

(continued)

Figure 2-5

Traditionally, Hindus undergo cremation after the body has ceased to function, and they believe in the reincarnation of the spirit into the next life. The family of the young man wanted to follow those traditions. They needed to be able to scatter the child's ashes on sacred ground, the Ganges River in India. Wanting the family to have this final request, the two students and I got to work. Preparing the body for transport to India would have been difficult and very expensive. However, working with a local funeral home, the two students were able to properly prepare and view the body before cremation and participate in their traditional chanting and prayers for the dead. Pictures of the young man were taken, and the cremation was completed. The ashes and pictures were then sent to India, where the parents could perform the traditional Hindu ceremonies, burn the pictures of their child, and scatter his ashes in their final tribute.

With the efforts of a good nursing assessment, the Hindu circle of life had been completed. The life of this young man had been short but strived toward perfection within a religion that dates back 5,000 years; his soul had been released and removed from the confines of his current life and had the ability to move forward into the next realm. As a nurse, I was moved and forever changed.

R. Peterson, RN, MSN

Figure 2-5 (Continued)

ASSESSMENT: THE MANAGED CARE ENVIRONMENT

Today's health care environment has necessitated additions to the nursing history that the nurse completes. The additions include relating the individualized patient assessment to the case management plan and consideration of the resources of the patient that should be utilized in meeting health care needs.

Case Management Plan

The case management plan may take the form of a critical pathway that has been developed by a multidisciplinary team. Expert nurse clinicians who have cared for many patients with a specific medical diagnosis have worked together with other health care team members to determine a generic "admission to discharge" plan of patient care. These expert nurses, using their experience, have identified the high frequency problems associated with a given medical diagnosis. The registered nurse who admits the patient will complete an assessment and determine

whether there is a preexisting critical pathway that will meet the needs of the patient. Often the case manager makes this initial assessment in a preoperative clinic before surgery and begins the critical pathway at that time. At other times the case manager may work with the registered nurse on staff to validate the correct placement on a critical pathway and assist in the modification of that pathway to meet individual needs. It is also the responsibility of the admitting nurse to begin to individualize the care of a patient placed on a generic critical pathway.

The case manager or staff nurse also begins discharge planning at this initial contact with patients and families. Many institutions do not implement discharge planning but have chosen to use the term *transition planning*. This term recognizes that patients often require additional care in a different setting after leaving the hospital. Patients may be admitted to a nursing home for a period of time to receive skilled nursing care until they are able to return home. Other patients may receive care at home. Here care may include nursing care as well as social work services, nutritional support, physical therapy, and occupational therapy or home infusion therapies. All this care must be carefully coordinated and individualized to meet patients' needs.

While it may be impossible to know with certainty what care will be needed upon discharge from the hospital, experienced nurses can identify cues in the admission history. For example, consider the case of an elderly patient who lives alone and has had hip replacement therapy. The nurse can begin to talk with the patient about planning for home care. The nurse might introduce the topic by saying, "I have cared for many patients who have had this surgery. They usually need assistance at home for a time. Have you thought about how you can manage at home?" This will give the patient the opportunity to confirm that help may be needed or that plans already have been made. Often the nurse may find that while an elderly patient is in the hospital, family members express concern that it is no longer safe for the patient to live independently or that they are no longer able to care for the patient. This is a very complex situation requiring careful assessment and validation of the patient's needs and wishes. It also requires skilled communication with all family members.

Of course, not all institutions have case managers. These coordination and planning functions are then within the role of staff nurses. In this case staff nurses need to be well informed about the institutional resources available to them. The staff nurse may request a consultation from a clinical social worker to assist with nursing home placement. Home health agencies have intake nurses who assess whether the patient is eligible for home nursing care. An often overlooked member of the team is a physical therapist who will be able to complete a safety assessment of the patient's home and determine ongoing physical therapy needs. A careful and up-to-date assessment of the patient's needs and resources will assure that advance planning can be completed successfully. Discharge planning that begins at discharge is likely to be fragmented and incomplete and often causes costly delays.

Assessment of Health Care Resources

Another important part of the nursing assessment is an investigation of the resources that the patient has to commit to health care. Probably the most obvious question is: Does the patient have health insurance, and if so, what is covered? If patients are over 65 years of age, they may have Medicare. Because Medicare is changing so rapidly, the nurse may consult the Internet for the most current documents concerning Medicare coverage. The site address is http://www.medicare.gov/. On this site it is possible to find Spanish and Asian-language translations as well as the English version. The nurse also may call 1-800-MEDICARE for information. Many persons who have Medicare insurance carry a Medicare supplement for the things that Medicare does not cover, such as prescription drugs. Some Medicare patients have enrolled in health maintenance organizations (HMOs). This type of insurance coverage usually requires preapproval to assure payment of covered expenses. Payment for Medicaid programs that cover low-income persons varies from state to state. It is very appropriate for the nurse to call the insurance company and ask about the extent of coverage. However, before the nurse communicates with the insurance company, it is essential that there be a signed authorization from the patient for release of information to insurance companies in the medical record. To discuss a patient without this signed release is a violation of confidentiality and a violation of both legal rights and professional ethics. There are two particular patients' situations that require specific authorization for the release of information. Persons with AIDS and persons with a psychiatric illness are protected from violations of confidentiality. Most states require specific authorizations for the release of this information. It is not unusual for these patients to choose to pay for the costs of hospitalization and treatment themselves rather than release information about the illness to an insurance company.

There are many other sources of financial aid available to patients. It is genuinely helpful to patients if the nurse is able to discuss those sources and assist patients in obtaining aid. Often a clinical social worker is a resource for the nurse in this area or is the team member responsible for matching resources to need.

While insurance is an important area of the assessment of resources, the nurse also considers the availability of people to help the patient at home as another resource in discharge planning. Consider whether family members live near enough to be helpful. Is there a caregiver in the home, or does the patient live alone? Increasingly, nurses may observe that the patient is the caregiver for an elderly spouse and that the spouse may require assistance while the caregiver recovers. If a child is the patient, the nurse assesses whether the parents are available to provide care after discharge or if their work schedules necessitate other arrangements. The nurse needs to remain nonjudgmental, especially in the case of parents who are unable to stay home and care for their children. Perhaps the income from both jobs is essential to providing food and shelter for the family even though the parents would choose to be home if they could.

Other areas of resource assessment include availability of transportation for follow-up care, meal preparation and grocery shopping, safety of the home environment with special consideration to bathroom facilities, access to emergency assistance (for example, the nearness of the telephone to the patient's bedroom, and the ability to understand self-care teaching).

Following the customer service approach of other industries, some hospitals have initiated the practice of telephone follow-up calls after discharge for each patient within 24 to 72 hours. This provides another opportunity for the nurse to assess the patient and identify actual or potential problems.

SUMMARY

Assessment is the first step in the nursing process and the one step that is a part of every other step in the nursing process. The nursing assessment that the nurse completes upon the patient's admission to the hospital focuses on the patient's response to actual or potential health problems. During assessment the nurse collects data by interview, observation, examination, and medical record review. The nurse does not make judgments or conclusions at this time but focuses on establishing a comprehensive data base that reflects the health status of the patient. Similarly, the nurse seeks to gather only data, not judgments and conclusions, from the patient through the use of open questions: "What is your normal pattern of . . .? Has it changed with illness? Are you doing anything to cope with the changes?"

PRACTICE EXERCISE

I. Consider the following pieces of data and label them:

O = objective
S = subjective
J = judgment or conclusions.

1. 75 cc dark amber urine.
2 Patient is afraid of surgery because her mother died in the hospital.
3. "I can't go that long (8 hours) without smoking."
4. Large amount of bright red drainage from incision site.
5. Patient states that the pain is 8 on 1–10 scale.
6. Respiratory rate of 36 after walking length of hall unassisted.
7. Patient's oral intake is in excess of body requirements.
8. Intelligent and articulate middle-aged adult.

9. Confused elderly white male.
10. Patient is becoming increasingly agitated.

II. Given the following patient responses, formulate two additional questions the nurse might ask that would encourage the patient to provide more complete information about his or her response to actual or high-risk health problems.

1. Patient is an 86-year-old woman with arthritis who lives alone in her own home. You are to assess her mobility status.
NURSE: "Do you have any problems getting around?"
PATIENT: "Nope."

2. Patient is a 12-year-old boy with possible appendicitis. You are to assess pain.
NURSE: "Are you having any pain?"
PATIENT: "No—can I go home now?"

3. Patient is a 45-year-old woman who is slightly overweight. You are to assess the client's nutritional status.
NURSE: "Do you have any nutritional problems?"
PATIENT: "None other than eating too much."

4. Patient is a 53-year-old man admitted for a possible heart attack. You are to assess the patient's coping skills/stress management.
NURSE: "Do you feel that you are under a lot of stress?"
PATIENT: "No more than most people."

5. Patient is a 17-year-old high school football team captain admitted for diagnostic tests for mononucleosis. You are initiating the nursing assessment.
NURSE: "How have you been feeling?"
PATIENT: "Not too bad."

ANSWERS TO EXERCISE ON ASSESSMENT

I.

1. O
2. J
3. S
4. J (Use of word *large* makes it a judgment.)
5. S

6. O
7. J
8. J
9. J (Describe the behaviors that made you label the patient as confused. State the patient's age.)
10. J (Describe the behaviors that made you label the patient as agitated.)

II.

1. "Can you tell me how you manage things such as cooking and grocery shopping?"
   "Has your arthritis made this hard for you to do?"
   "What things have you figured out that help you?"
2. "It sounds like you want to get out of here. Have you ever been in a hospital before?"
   "What was that like for you?"
   "What did the nurses do then that helped you?"
   "Do you think that if your side stops hurting you can go home?"
3. "What would be a typical breakfast, lunch, supper for you?"
   "What do you like for snacks"?
   "Are you able to exercise?"
4. "How much stress is normal for 'most people'?"
   "How do you cope with stress?"
   "Does it work for you?"
5. "What is 'not too bad' for you?"
   "And what do you do when you feel like that?"
   "Does that help?"
   "What problems brought you into the hospital or to the doctor?"

CASE STUDY: ASSESSMENT

The case study method will be used throughout this book to illustrate the steps in the nursing process. In any clinical setting in which the nurse cares for patients, the nursing process is used to plan and evaluate nursing care. This case study will illustrate how nurses in four settings across the care continuum use the nursing process. The patient in this case study is *first* seen in an orthopedic surgery clinic. Patients have been referred to the clinic by their own primary care physicians for possible orthopedic surgery. The *second* setting is a first day surgery center. Patients are admitted to this center on the morning of surgery for their scheduled procedures. After the surgical procedures, they are transferred to the inpatient nursing unit for their hospital stay. The *third* setting is the orthopedic postoperative patient care unit in the hospital. The *fourth* setting is the patient's home, where the nurse is an employee of a home health care agency.

Each care plan begins with a nursing assessment that builds on the data collected by the nurse in the previous setting. Each nurse is accountable for reviewing the documentation of the assessment and plan of care completed by the previous nurse. The student may study the care plan by reading the complete care plan of the previous nurse in one setting, moving from chapter to chapter. A second approach is to study the steps of the process as illustrated by four nurses who each complete one step of the process in a different care setting.

The case study of Mrs. Wiley will be found in each chapter. Mrs. Wiley was seen in the orthopedic surgery clinic, where she was referred by her family physician. She has been complaining of knee pain for several years that has become progressively worse in the last 9 months.

NURSING ASSESSMENT #1

Preoperative Orthopedic Surgery Clinic

(Data Collection Format based on Maslow's basic needs framework)

General Information

Information given by: patient   Today's date: 10/17/00

Name: Mrs. William (Jennifer) Wiley

Age: 74 years   Sex: female   Race: Caucasian

Date of scheduled surgery: 10/29/00

Scheduled admission: 10/29/00   Time: 0600

Surgical procedure: total knee arthroplasty, right knee

Insurance coverage: Medicare with Service Plus supplement. Patient states, "Finances are not a concern. We both have a pension and substantial savings. If we need to pay something by ourselves, that is okay."

Vital signs: T. 98.6, P. 84, R. 22, BP 136/90, weight 156, height 5'5", Pain: 6

Advanced directives: completed and updated within last year. Copy with husband, daughter, and primary care provider.

Patient's perception of surgery: "I need to have my knee joint replaced. I have been trying to avoid it, but now the pain is too much and I have to have it done. I have never been in the hospital except for my maternity stay. I have no idea what to expect."

How has the problem been managed at home? "I try to stay off it as much as possible, but I like to play golf and really cannot do that due to the pain. I take Motrin or Tylenol for the pain, but lately that doesn't help."

Allergies: no known allergies
_____

Medications: Tylenol or Motrin over the counter for pain; no prescription meds
_____

Physiological Needs

OXYGENATION: nonsmoker all her life; respirations 22, lungs clear, no cough, no complaints of dyspnea on movement; pulse 84, strong and regular; no heart murmurs, denies any chest pain; 2- to 3-second capillary refill of fingernail beds; no ankle or leg edema; skin pink and slightly dry.

TEMPERATURE MAINTENANCE: T. 98.6; denies any fever in last 2 weeks; states, "I am rarely sick."

NUTRITIONAL–FLUID: weight 156, height 5'5"; reports good appetite; has maintained same weight over last 10 years; no known food allergies; goes out to lunch two to three times per week with friends.

ELIMINATION.   last bowel movement 10/16; normal pattern qod; denies stool is hard or difficult to pass; occasionally takes a laxative at bedtime if necessary; no problems with urination, though some stress incontinence with coughing or sneezing.

REST–SLEEP: sleeps 6 to 7 hours per night; may nap in the afternoon; no use of sleeping pills.

PAIN AVOIDANCE: rates knee pain as a 6 on a scale of 1–10; states, "When it is bad, the Tylenol doesn't touch it anymore. It really interferes with the things I enjoy doing."

SEXUALITY–REPRODUCTIVE: lives with 80-year-old husband who is frail and weak; "I don't know what he would do without me. He can't cook for himself or really be safe overnight alone. What if he falls?"; has never been in the hospital with the exception of childbirth; two children, ages 42 (son) and 35 (daughter), both living out of state.

STIMULATION–ACTIVITY: college graduate; speaks fluent Spanish; enjoys friends, playing cards, and water aerobics; spends afternoons at senior center with her husband and friends; she drives during the day; her husband no longer drives.

Safety–Security Needs

She is alert and oriented; mini-mental status score of 30 (no cognitive impairment); good vision with bifocals.

Love–Belonging Needs

Mrs. Wiley has been married for 48 years; she describes her husband as "all right as long as I am there to look after him. That is the problem when I have to be in the hospital: Who will do for him?"

Self-Esteem Needs

"I need to be able to get my work done and help my husband. I cannot live like an invalid or a frail old lady dependent on others for everything."

Self-Actualization Needs

"We have a wonderful life, full of friends and enjoying our children and grand-children."

NURSING ASSESSMENT #2

First Day Surgery Unit: 6 A.M.

Information given by: patient   Today's Date: 10/29/00

Name: Mrs. William (Jennifer) Wiley

Time of admission: 0600

Surgical procedure: total knee arthroplasty, right knee

Vital signs: T. 98.8, P. 88, R. 26, BP 138/90, no pain at present, weight 156, height 5′5″

Advanced directives: copy in chart

Patient's perception of surgery: "The clinic nurse taught me about the surgery. I have practiced crutch walking but don't feel comfortable with it yet. The home health nurse came out to check the house and make sure it was safe for me after surgery."

How has the problem been managed at home? "My daughter will stay with my husband until I get home, but I am afraid. What if the surgery makes it worse? I need to able to help my husband."

Allergies: no known allergies

Medications: currently taking no prescription pain medications; Motrin/Tylenol for pain; none for last week

Home health nurse note: six steps into home from front door, two if entered via attached garage; wall-to-wall carpet with exception of kitchen; small area rugs removed; first floor bathroom and bedroom; will arrange to add railings to tub/shower, bench in bathtub at safe height and stable.

Physiological Needs

OXYGENATION: Respirations 26, lungs clear, no cough, no complaints of dyspnea on movement; pulse 88, strong and regular; no heart murmurs, denies any chest pain; 2- to 3-second capillary refill of fingernail beds; no ankle or leg edema; skin pink and slightly dry.

MOBILITY: physical therapy noted that Mrs. Wiley will need additional instruction in crutch walking after surgery; has difficulty manipulating crutches on stairs.

TEMPERATURE MAINTENANCE: T. 98.6; denies any fever in last 2 weeks.

NUTRITIONAL–FLUID: weight 156, height 5′5″

ELIMINATION: last bowel movement 10/29, soft and formed; urine specimen to lab.

REST–SLEEP: slept 6 hours last night

PAIN AVOIDANCE: no pain at present

SAFETY–SECURITY: shakiness, jitters of hands (Mrs. W.), trembling voice (daughter and husband), darting eye movements (husband)

SEXUALITY–REPRODUCTIVE: accompanied by daughter and husband

SAFETY–SECURITY NEEDS: alert and oriented; mini-mental status score of 30 (no cognitive impairment); bifocals with daughter until after surgery.

NURSING ASSESSMENT #3

Postoperative Orthopedic Patient Care Unit

Date: 10/29/00   Time: 1:00 P.M. (1300)

Time	Temp	Pulse	Resp	BP	Pain rating
1300	98.2/36.8	88	20	130/84	6
1400		94	20	136/88	8

10/29/00 1300 admission note:

Admitted to unit from recovery room. Sedated but arousable. IV D5/.45 NS c̄ 20 KCL @100 cc/h. Elastic stocking to nonoperative leg. Operative leg elevated, and knee in full extension. Morphine PCA to right forearm. Operative dressing clean and dry; 80 cc drainage in constavac. Skin warm and dry. Oriented patient and family to room, food service, and nursing staff. Reinforced PCA teaching. Husband cried on wife's return from surgery. Appears tired and states that he "worried a lot last night and not much sleep. We've been together 52 years now. Nothing is right when my Jenny isn't home." Daughter reports father unable to eat and increasingly irritable, "which is not his normal self." Aware of physical therapy notes that Mrs. Wiley was having difficulty preop with crutch walking.

_____

(signature)

10/29/00 1400 nursing note:

Reinforced teaching re PCA. Repositioned. States, "I feel like a dishrag—can't even move in bed by myself, but I am so glad that it is over." Needs assistance to turn and reposition in bed. IV site intact—no redness, pain, swelling. Able to deep breathe with coaching. Unable to use incentive spirometer yet. Taking sips; no nausea reported.

_____

(signature)

NURSING ASSESSMENT #4

Home Health Care Agency

Mrs. Wiley: The nurse caring for Mrs. Wiley on the postoperative orthopedic unit has made a referral to the home health agency as part of the discharge or

transition planning process. Part 1 was completed by the intake nurse from the agency while Mrs. Wiley was in the hospital. Part 2 is the skilled nursing assessment completed by the registered nurse in the home at the time of the first visit.

Part 1

PATIENT GENERAL INFORMATION Patient name: Jennifer Wiley SS Number: 395-99-1873 Phone: 920-571-8241 Address: 3401 Elmwood Place City: Madison, State: WI ZIP 60823	DIRECTIONS: Main Street south to Hwy. 63 east for 3 miles. Exit at Lakeland and turn right 6 blocks to turn right on Elmwood. White house with blue shutters.
HAZARD AREA: none	PAYER SOURCE: Medicare with Service Plus supplement
Room Number: University Hospital 6-741	Physician: Dr. A. Harker MD 920-864-8254 Medical Diagnosis: Osteoarthritis NOS*; orthopedic aftercare NOS
Referral Log Comment: total knee arthroplasty Anticipated discharge date: 11/02/00	Surgical Procedure: Total knee replacement
DATE OF BIRTH: 10/18/26 AGE: 74 years RACE: Caucasian SEX: F Marital Status: M Lives alone (Y/N): N	
EMERGENCY CONTACT: William Wiley (husband): 920-571-8241 Susan Wiley Thurston (daughter): 517-933-8734	
ACCEPTED TO SERVICE: Susan Jaily, RN	

* NOS = not otherwise specified.

Part 2 Visit date: 11/03/00   10:34 A.M.

REASON FOR HOME CARE: Orthopedic aftercare. Needs physical therapy for assisted ambulation and gait training, ROM and upper body strengthening. Assessment of incision, med management, pain management, functional safety, and safety in home.

CLINICAL ASSESSMENT: 10:34 A.M.

TEMPERATURE: 97.6 F (36.4 C) Pulse: 88 radial regular BP: 138/80 Weight: 155 pounds

NUTRITION: states, "I'm really tired and not much of an appetite."

EDEMA: right lower extremity, #2 from foot to knee

PAIN: rt knee, severity 3 to 4. Took one Tylenol #3 11:30 A.M. States, "It is less painful if I just stay put and do not move."

ORIENTATION: oriented to time, person, place; cooperative.

MOBILITY: decreased mobility and activity. "I was in too much pain in the hospital to really work at it. It is one thing to do it with the therapist in the hospital, but my home is carpeted and a lot trickier. I really feel safer with a walker." PT will assess later today. Order for weight bearing as tolerated.

SKIN: warm and dry.

WOUND: rt. knee. Linear incision intact with staples.

LEARNING NEEDS/SELF-CARE: "They talked about all that while I was in the hospital, but I was too scared to absorb it."

LIVING SITUATION: Meals-on-Wheels to start this A.M. 2 × day. Husband provides limited assistance with household tasks. Neighbors and daughter to check in daily.

HEAD AND NECK: vision—needs glasses at all times.

MEDICATIONS:
Tylenol #3, 1 or 2 q4h prn
Metamucil—patient takes as she decides
Multivitamin—1 per day OTC
Ibuprofen OTC as necessary.

SAFETY: clear path to bathroom, raised toilet seat, no tub railings; no throw rugs; attached garage, first floor bedroom, bed immobile.

Diagnosis

Diagnosis is the second step in the nursing process and is the phase during which the nurse analyzes the data gathered during assessment and identifies problem areas for the patient. The nurse then makes a nursing diagnosis. The terms *nursing diagnosis* and *diagnosing* do not mean the same thing in this chapter and may be confusing for the student. *Diagnosing* is a process of data analysis and problem identification. It is a form of decision making that the nurse uses to arrive at judgments and conclusions about patients' responses to actual or potential health problems. A *nursing diagnosis* is the specific result of diagnosing and is the problem statement that nurses use to communicate professionally. It refers to a problem statement that the nurse makes regarding a patient's condition. The American Nurses Association (ANA) defines nursing diagnosis as a clinical judgment about the patient's response to actual or potential health conditions or needs (1998). It is helpful to think of these terms as a noun (nursing diagnosis) or verb (diagnose) to distinguish between the two. The purpose of the nursing diagnosis is to "provide the basis for determination of a plan of care to achieve expected outcomes" (ANA, 1998) for a patient's health status.

There are three activities in the diagnosis step:

$$\text{Diagnosing} = \text{Data Analysis} + \text{Problem Identification} + \text{Formulation of Nursing Diagnosis}$$

DATA ANALYSIS

QUESTION: "So now that I've got all these data, what do I do with them?"
ANSWER: "Make sense out of them and use them."

The nurse has completed the initial systematic data collection and is now ready to begin the process of analysis. The nurse begins the activity of data analysis by considering all the data that were gathered during the assessment phase of the nursing process. The nurse quickly checks for completeness of the data. For example, if the data were collected in a format that used Maslow's hierarchy of basic needs, data about rest and sleep patterns may be unclear, incomplete, or omitted. The nurse may decide to go back and gather additional data as needed.

Another aspect of completeness is the cultural context of the data. While it may be difficult for nurses to go beyond the perspective of their own cultures, it is essential to analyze the data within the context of the culture of the patient. An example of this is a consideration of how pain is expressed within various cultures. Some cultures are open in expressing pain, while others place a high value on stoicism and self-control. It is necessary for the nurse to be sensitive to the culture of the patient and to assure that data collection includes the patient's cultural uniqueness. See the section on Culturally Competent Nursing Care During Diagnosis later in this chapter.

The nurse also looks for inconsistencies or ambiguity in the data. It may become apparent to the nurse that the sequence of events in the history is contradictory and needs to be resolved. Two data sources may be inconsistent. For example, the patient may report having only an occasional "social drink," while the spouse gives data about "drinking 10 to 12 cans of beer daily." At this point no judgment is made about the existence of a problem, but the inconsistency is noted. Another example might be that the nurse does not understand from reading the assessment what methods the patient has used for pain relief and with what result.

The data are evaluated for comprehensiveness: Do the data give a complete picture of the patient, considering both physical and psychosocial aspects of the person? The nurse asks whether the assessment has considered all areas that may be relevant to the patient. This considers things such as higher level needs, cultural factors, and data related to growth and development in addition to the more obvious physical areas. These factors taken together constitute holistic health, that is, the concept that the mind and the body are inseparable and that one cannot be treated without the other. In summary, the nurse reviews the data for clarity, consistency, completeness, and comprehensiveness.

After reviewing the data, the nurse continues analysis by studying the data and making judgments and conclusions about the meaning of the data. The nurse will decide if the data indicate a problem for the patient, or a situation that puts the patient at risk for the development of problems in the future. The following decisions are based on the data:

1. Determine whether measurement data are within the normal range for the patient and within the norms for that patient's age group. For example, if the nurse has taken the blood pressure (BP) of the patient, the nurse can now ask if this pressure is typical for this individual. The nurse also determines if this BP reading is within the normal range for this patient's age.
2. Determine if the functioning described by the patient is typical of past functioning and within normal patterns for the patient's age. The nurse could consider the bowel elimination pattern that the patient reported as "every other day, soft and easy to pass, no blood, no use of laxatives but daily bran flakes, no change with diabetes" and decide that the pattern is both typical for the patient and within normal patterns for adults.
3. Determine what relationships exist between pieces of data. For example, if the data reveal that the patient is 25% overweight, has elevated blood pressure, and has no understanding of caloric content of food and body requirements, the nurse recognizes the relationship between the many factors that affect the obesity. Another patient may be unable to sleep, appear very anxious, be very demanding of the nurses' time, and have a history that includes a parent who died during a routine surgical procedure. While the obvious interpretation that the patient is also worried about dying during surgery needs confirmation by the patient, it seems clear that there is a relationship between the data.
4. Evaluate the physical assessment data as positive, negative, normal, or abnormal signs or findings. For example, if the nurse has completed auscultation of the patient's lungs, the nurse makes a decision if the findings were normal or not, and if not, which abnormality was heard and the location of the abnormal sound. This is clearly recorded. Similarly, the decision that a particular aspect of the examination was negative is valuable because it notes that a judgment has been made and a problem has been ruled out. These decisions may be difficult for a beginning nurse to make. Until the nurse has had a lot of experience, it is difficult to judge what are normal versus abnormal lung sounds. The student should not hesitate to ask a more experienced nurse to assist in this evaluation.
5. Determine whether specific behavior patterns contribute to the health and well-being of the patient. The nurse may evaluate that the dietary and exercise patterns of the patient foster cardiovascular health as in the case of the patient who reports that she has never smoked, has decreased her intake of red meat to twice a week, and walks 2 miles a day several times a week. The nurse considers the opposite decision in the case of the patient who reports that she is a pack-a-day smoker, "My father died of a heart attack," needs to lose 30 pounds, and has no physical activity. Here the nurse would also try to determine if the patient perceives these things to be problematic and is willing to make any life-style changes. While the nurse may evaluate something to be a problem, the adult patient always has the right to make a decision to refuse the health professional's recommendations. Although this may generate feelings of ineffectiveness and frustration in the nurse, it is the goal of health education to assist patients in making informed decisions, and

it is the right of patients to make decisions within the context of their own values, beliefs, and culture.

6. Determine the strengths and resources as well as limitations of the patients as they affect health status. These may include things such as cognitive abilities or potential, willingness to change, family support, economic resources, and available time to invest. For example, a nursing student who is going to school full-time and working part-time probably would have little time, energy, or money to invest in an exercise club. For another patient, the nurse may make the judgment that the YMCA membership the patient holds is a valuable resource affecting health status. Another patient who has suffered a mild heart attack may state, "That was a warning. Now I am ready to do whatever I have to, to get healthy and stay healthy." The nurse may interpret that as a willingness to receive health teaching and a motivation to follow through.

PROBLEM IDENTIFICATION

The next step is to identify a broad focus area requiring nursing intervention, such as nutrition, elimination, or incorrect or inadequate information. This is the identification of a problem area. Nurses use nursing theory, general knowledge base, and cumulative experience to define this area. For example, in a patient who is a newly diagnosed Type 2 diabetic, the nurse may read data that include things such as a history of being overweight since childhood, "My mother used to bake me a chocolate whipped cream cake if I got a good report card," "I've tried every diet in the book," "I don't feel jolly—aren't fat people supposed to be jolly?" "My children are plump, but it is just baby fat and they'll grow out of it," patient is 43 years old, 5'2", weight 189 lbs. The nurse uses knowledge of human growth and development, behavioral psychology, anatomy and physiology, and nursing in considering these data. A focus for nursing intervention in the area of nutrition is indicated.

In a second example, another patient may include the following data: pain in the lower back, unable to perform job (cashier in a grocery store) because it causes pain, unable to do any housework without aggravation of pain, "I'm no use to anybody," "My mother had a bad back and was an invalid at age 45." Here the nurse also uses knowledge of sciences related to nursing to recognize that the data indicate an area for nursing intervention. The nurse identifies the back pain as the most immediate problem focus area requiring intervention, although there are data to indicate that the patient also is experiencing low self-esteem.

After a broad focus area is chosen, a narrower, more specific problem statement is selected from the diagnostic statements developed by the North American Nursing Diagnosis Association (NANDA).

NURSING DIAGNOSIS:

is a clinical judgment about the client's response to actual or potential health conditions or needs. (ANA, 1998)

At this point the student may choose to consult the *Nursing Diagnosis Pocketbook* that is included with this text. Table 3-1 lists the problem focus areas corresponding to basic human needs. Specific nursing diagnoses developed by NANDA are listed under each focus area. Alternatively, the student may use Table 3-2, which is a listing of NANDA diagnostic categories. These categories are organized according to nine human response patterns as a broad focus area.

The next step in the process is to move from the completed data analysis with the identification of a focus area to the determination of the correct nursing diagnosis. Consider the following data that the nurse has documented from the admission nursing history of the patient Mrs. Jones:

—54 years old, has had three children
—complains of involuntary loss of urine "when I cough or sneeze or during exercise"
—"I have to go to the bathroom all the time—I can't sit through a movie without having to get up to use the rest room"

The nurse reviews the basic needs framework of Maslow and selects a focus area of *Elimination Needs*. Further review of the two major categories in this area indicates a choice between *Bowel* and *Urinary* elimination, and the nurse selects the subcategory *Urinary Elimination*. Nursing diagnoses under this category include

- Altered urinary elimination
- Functional urinary incontinence
- Reflex urinary incontinence
- Stress incontinence
- Toileting self-care deficit
- Total incontinence
- Risk for urinary urge incontinence
- Urge incontinence
- Urinary retention

The nurse can easily eliminate two diagnoses: toileting self-care deficit and urinary retention. Neither of these is related to the symptoms the patient has evidenced. Now the nurse uses a process of matching the patient's symptoms to the defining characteristics of the nursing diagnoses. For example, the nursing diagnosis of reflex incontinence has as defining characteristics no awareness of bladder filling and no urge to void or feelings of bladder fullness. Mrs. Jones has

TABLE 3-1   NURSING DIAGNOSES ORGANIZED BY BASIC HUMAN NEED

1. **Oxygen Needs**
   —Altered tissue perfusion (specify: renal, cerebral, cardiopulmonary, gastrointestinal, peripheral)
   —Decreased cardiac output
   —Dysfunctional ventilatory weaning response
   —Impaired gas exchange
   —Inability to sustain spontaneous ventilation
   —Ineffective airway clearance
   —Ineffective breathing pattern
   —Risk for aspiration
   —Risk for peripheral neurovascular dysfunction
   —Risk for suffocation
2. **Temperature Maintenance**
   —Hypothermia
   —Hyperthermia
   —Ineffective thermoregulation
   —Risk for altered body temperature
3. **Nutritional and Fluid Needs**
   —Altered nutrition: less than body requirements
   —Altered nutrition: more than body requirements
   —Altered nutrition: risk for more than body requirements
   —Altered dentition
   —Effective breast feeding
   —Ineffective breast feeding
   —Ineffective infant feeding pattern
   —Interrupted breast feeding
   —Feeding self-care deficit
   —Risk for fluid volume deficit
   —Fluid volume deficit
   —Fluid volume excess
   —Risk for fluid volume imbalance
   —Impaired swallowing
4. **Elimination Needs**
   Toileting self-care deficit
   Bowel
   　—Bowel incontinence
   　—Constipation
   　—Risk for constipation
   　—Perceived constipation
   　—Diarrhea
   Urinary
   　—Altered urinary elimination
   　—Functional urinary incontinence

  —Reflex urinary incontinence
  —Stress incontinence
  —Total incontinence
  —Risk for urinary urge incontinence
  —Urge incontinence
  —Urinary retention

5. **Rest and Sleep Needs**
  —Fatigue
  —Sleep pattern disturbance
  —Sleep deprivation

6. **The Need for Pain Avoidance**
  —Pain
  —Chronic pain
  —Nausea

7. **Sexual Needs**
  —Altered sexuality patterns
  —Sexual dysfunction

8. **Stimulation Needs**
  —Risk for activity intolerance
  —Activity intolerance
  —Diversional activity deficit
  —Impaired physical mobility
  —Risk for perioperative positioning injury
  —Impaired walking
  —Impaired wheelchair mobility
  —Impaired transfer ability
  —Impaired bed mobility
  —Risk for disuse syndrome
  —Sensory/perceptual alterations (specify: visual, auditory, kinesthetic, gustatory, tactile, olfactory)
  —Unilateral neglect

9. **Safety and Security Needs**
  Physiological level
  —Altered health maintenance
  —Altered oral mucous membrane
  —Altered protection
  —Risk for autonomic dysreflexia
  —Dysreflexia
  —Impaired home maintenance management
  —Risk for impaired skin integrity
  —Impaired skin integrity
  —Impaired tissue integrity
  —Risk for infection
  —Risk for injury
  —Risk for poisoning

—Risk for trauma
—Delayed surgical recovery
—Adult failure to thrive
—Altered growth and development
—Risk for altered development
—Risk for altered growth
—Risk for disorganized infant behavior
—Disorganized infant behavior
—Potential for enhanced organized infant behavior
—Latex allergy response
—Risk for latex allergy response
—Decreased adaptive capacity: intracranial
—Energy field disturbance
Higher level
—Altered thought processes
—Impaired environmental interpretation syndrome
—Acute confusion
—Chronic confusion
—Impaired memory
—Relocation stress syndrome

10. Love and Belonging Needs
—Altered family processes
—Altered family processes: alcoholism
—Risk for altered parent/infant/child attachment
—Risk for altered parenting
—Altered parenting
—Parental role conflict
—Risk for caregiver role strain
—Caregiver role strain
—Anticipatory grieving
—Dysfunctional grieving
—Impaired verbal communication
—Impaired social interaction
—Social isolation
—Risk for loneliness
—Chronic sorrow

11. Spiritual Needs
—Spiritual distress (distress of the human spirit)
—Risk for spiritual distress
—Potential for enhanced spiritual well-being
—Anxiety
—Death anxiety
—Decisional conflict (specify)
—Fear
—Ineffective denial

—Ineffective family coping: disabling
—Ineffective family coping: compromised
—Ineffective community coping
—Impaired adjustment
—Ineffective individual coping
—Ineffective management of therapeutic regimen: individual
—Ineffective management of therapeutic regimen: families
—Ineffective management of therapeutic regimen: community
—Effective management of therapeutic regimen: individual
—Knowledge deficit (specify)
—Noncompliance (specify)
—Risk for violence: self-directed
—Risk for violence: directed at others
—Risk for self-mutilation
—Risk for post-trauma syndrome
—Post-trauma syndrome
—Rape-trauma syndrome: compound reaction
—Rape-trauma syndrome: silent reaction

12. Self-Esteem
—Altered role performance
—Bathing/hygiene/self-care deficit
—Body image disturbance
—Chronic low self-esteem
—Defensive coping
—Dressing/grooming self-care deficit
—Hopelessness
—Personal identity disturbance
—Powerlessness
—Self-esteem disturbance
—Situational low self-esteem

13. Self-Actualization Needs
—Family coping: potential for growth
—Health-seeking behaviors (specify)
—Potential for enhanced community coping

Source: Adapted from *NANDA Nursing Diagnoses: Definitions and Classification 1999–2000.*
Philadelphia, North American Nursing Diagnosis Association, 1999, with permission.

complained of feeling frequent needs to void even at intervals of shorter duration than a movie. Thus, the nursing diagnosis of reflex incontinence is inaccurate. For the nursing diagnosis of stress incontinence, the defining characteristic
is reported dribbling of urine with increased abdominal pressure. Another characteristic is urinary frequency more often than every 2 hours. Both of these characteristics match the symptoms reported by Mrs. Jones, and the nurse may
reliably make the nursing diagnosis of stress incontinence.

TABLE 3-2   APPROVED NANDA NURSING DIAGNOSTIC CATEGORIES LISTED BY
HUMAN RESPONSE SYSTEM

Pattern 1: Exchanging
Altered nutrition: more than body requirements
Altered nutrition: less than body requirements
Altered nutrition: risk for more than body requirements
Risk for infection
Risk for altered body temperature
Hypothermia
Hyperthermia
Ineffective thermoregulation
Dysreflexia
Risk for autonomic dysreflexia
Constipation
Perceived constipation
Diarrhea
Bowel incontinence
Risk for constipation
Altered urinary elimination
Stress incontinence
Reflex urinary incontinence
Urge incontinence
Functional urinary incontinence
Total incontinence
Risk for urinary urge incontinence
Urinary retention
Altered tissue perfusion (specify: renal, cerebral, cardiopulmonary,
gastrointestinal, peripheral)
Risk for fluid volume imbalance
Fluid volume excess
Fluid volume deficit
Risk for fluid volume deficit
Decreased cardiac output
Impaired gas exchange
Ineffective airway clearance
Ineffective breathing pattern
Inability to sustain spontaneous ventilation
Dysfunctional ventilatory weaning response
Risk for injury
Risk for suffocation
Risk for poisoning
Risk for trauma
Risk for aspiration
Risk for disuse syndrome

Latex allergy response
Risk for latex allergy response
Altered protection
Impaired tissue integrity
Altered oral mucous membrane
Impaired skin integrity
Risk for impaired skin integrity
Altered dentition
Decreased adaptive capacity: intracranial
Energy field disturbance
Pattern 2: Communicating
Impaired verbal communication
Pattern 3: Relating
Impaired social interaction
Social isolation
Risk for loneliness
Altered role performance
Altered parenting
Risk for altered parenting
Risk for altered parent/infant/child attachment
Sexual dysfunction
Altered family processes
Caregiver role strain
Risk for caregiver role strain
Altered family processes: alcoholism
Parental role conflict
Altered sexuality patterns
Pattern 4: Valuing
Spiritual distress (distress of the human spirit)
Risk for spiritual distress
Potential for enhanced spiritual well-being
Pattern 5: Choosing
Ineffective individual coping
Impaired adjustment
Defensive coping
Ineffective denial
Ineffective family coping: disabling
Ineffective family coping: compromised
Family coping: potential for growth
Potential for enhanced community coping
Ineffective community coping
Ineffective management of therapeutic regimen: individuals
Noncompliance (specify)
Ineffective management of therapeutic regimen: families
Ineffective management of therapeutic regimen: community

Effective management of therapeutic regimen: individual
Decisional conflict (specify)
Health-seeking behaviors (specify)
Pattern 6: Moving
Impaired physical mobility
Risk for peripheral neurovascular dysfunction
Risk for perioperative positioning injury
Impaired walking
Impaired wheelchair mobility
Impaired transfer ability
Impaired bed mobility
Activity intolerance
Fatigue
Risk for activity intolerance
Sleep pattern disturbance
Sleep deprivation
Diversional activity deficit
Impaired home maintenance management
Altered health maintenance
Delayed surgical recovery
Adult failure to thrive
Feeding self-care deficit
Impaired swallowing
Ineffective breast feeding
Interrupted breast feeding
Effective breast feeding
Ineffective infant feeding pattern
Bathing/hygiene self-care deficit
Dressing/grooming self-care deficit
Toileting self-care deficit
Altered growth and development
Risk for altered development
Risk for altered growth
Relocation stress syndrome
Risk for disorganized infant behavior
Disorganized infant behavior
Potential for enhanced organized infant behavior
Pattern 7: Perceiving
Body image disturbance
Self-esteem disturbance
Chronic low self-esteem
Situational low self-esteem
Personal identity disturbance
Sensory/perceptual alterations (specify: visual, auditory, kinesthetic,
gustatory, tactile, olfactory)

Unilateral neglect
Hopelessness
Powerlessness
Pattern 8: Knowing
Knowledge deficit (specify)
Impaired environmental interpretation syndrome
Acute confusion
Chronic confusion
Altered thought processes
Impaired memory
Pattern 9: Feeling
Pain
Chronic pain
Nausea
Dysfunctional grieving
Anticipatory grieving
Chronic sorrow
Risk for violence: directed at others
Risk for self-mutilation
Risk for violence: self-directed
Post-trauma syndrome
Rape-trauma syndrome
Rape-trauma syndrome: compound reaction
Rape-trauma syndrome: silent reaction
Anxiety
Death anxiety
Fear

Source: *NANDA Nursing Diagnoses: Definitions and Classification 1999–2000.* Philadelphia, North American Nursing Diagnosis Association, 1999, with permission.

FORMULATING THE NURSING DIAGNOSIS

The final activity in the process of diagnosing is the formulation of the nursing diagnosis.

The definition of a nursing diagnosis states that the problems the nurse chooses to address are within the scope of the legal practice of nursing, since this assumption underlies all professional activity. The privileges granted by licensure vary from state to state and country to country. Nurses with advanced degrees may be licensed to perform additional nursing care. However, all professional nurses share the responsibility for making nursing diagnoses within their practice.

A nursing diagnosis is not the same as a medical diagnosis, though it may involve the medical diagnosis or treatment as a cause. For example, the nursing

diagnosis of *pain* is clearly related to the medical diagnosis in many cases: Pain may be caused by a surgical incision, cancer that has metastasized to the bones, or stones in the gallbladder. However, since nurses cannot treat the medical diagnosis, the direction for nursing diagnosis must come from the problem part of the statement. Table 3-3 clarifies nursing diagnoses. A medical diagnosis frequently suggests nursing diagnoses. An experienced nurse who has cared for several patients with the same medical diagnosis will be able to predict some frequently occurring nursing diagnoses for a given medical condition. The nurse is then looking for data to validate the prediction. This experience contributes to skill in making nursing diagnoses. Table 3-4 gives examples of nursing diagnoses that are suggested by medical diagnoses.

The nurse begins the process of writing nursing diagnoses by reviewing the problem focus area identified in the previous step. Does the focus area represent a problem? By definition, a diagnosis must be a problem for the patient. If it is not a problem, no diagnosis need be made. Consider the bowel function status of a patient restricted to bed rest. If the patient has a soft, formed stool without exertion every 2 or 3 days, elimination is not a problem and no nursing diagnosis need be made. However, the nurse also considers who defines the problem. If the patient considers it abnormal not to have a bowel movement daily and continues to express anxiety related to this situation, a problem does exist as defined by the patient. The nurse understands that physiologically no problem exists but that the patient could benefit from teaching regarding normal body function. Nursing care may then focus on teaching as an intervention tool to reduce anxiety. Nursing diagnoses also may identify growth areas for the patient. Many nurses in industrial health or occupational health nursing report that the patients they see are requesting ways to improve their health status. While this does not constitute a problem, it is a focus area for nursing intervention. Tripp and Stachowiak (1989) proposed a nursing diagnosis that labels this as "health-seeking behavior." This nursing diagnosis does clearly identify an area of nursing intervention that is not a problem in the negative sense.

Types of Nursing Diagnoses

ACTUAL NURSING DIAGNOSES.   As defined here, the problem expressed in the nursing diagnosis may be either actual or at risk of occurring. An *actual nursing diagnosis* refers to a problem that exists at the present moment, in reality

TABLE 3-3   A NURSING DIAGNOSIS

Is	Is Not
A statement of a patient problem	A medical diagnosis
Actual, high risk, or possible	A nursing action
Within the scope of nursing practice	A physician order
Directive of nursing intervention	A therapeutic treatment

TABLE 3-4   MEDICAL DIAGNOSES THAT SUGGEST NURSING DIAGNOSES

Medical Diagnosis	Nursing Diagnosis
Myocardial infarction	Fear related to possible recurrence and uncertain outcome
Chronic ulcerative colitis	Diarrhea related to CUC as manifested by 10–12 loose, watery, foul-smelling stools per day
Chronic ulcerative colitis	Alteration in nutrition: less than body requirements related to altered GI absorption secondary to CUC
Cancer of the breast	High risk for body image disturbance if mastectomy is required
Cerebral vascular accident	Self-care deficit: dressing and grooming related to right-sided flaccidity

(Carroll-Johnson, 1991). A patient on a general diet with a good appetite has not had a bowel movement for 4 days, complains of low abdominal pain, and is unable to pass stool. The patient is constipated and requires nursing assistance. This situation requires that an actual nursing diagnosis be made.

RISK NURSING DIAGNOSES.   A *risk nursing diagnosis* is a clinical judgment that an individual, family, or community is more vulnerable to develop the problem than are others in the same or a similar situation. The nurse has identified factors in the admission data base or in ongoing assessments that indicate risk factors for the development of a problem. If a patient is on bed rest after total hip replacement, complains of pain on movement, and is poorly nourished, the patient is at risk for skin breakdown (decubitus ulcers). Understanding the physiological effect of prolonged bed rest, the nurse will implement interventions to prevent skin breakdown. In this example, the problem is one that requires preventive nursing action. The at-risk nursing diagnosis is based on the nurse's learning and past experience in similar situations and on an understanding of pathophysiology. The problem would predictably occur without nursing intervention. Nurses may choose to use "at risk" or "high risk" depending on the vulnerability of the patient (Carpenito, 1997).

POSSIBLE NURSING DIAGNOSES.   In still other situations the nurse may decide to formulate a tentative or *possible nursing diagnosis*. This may be compared to a physician who lists several "rule out" medical diagnoses in a patient's admission assessment. The physician may then order diagnostic tests to gather more data to make a decision. So it is with a possible nursing diagnoses. By considering a possible nursing diagnosis, the nurse assures the continued collection of relevant data. With an increased data base, the nurse may be able to firmly establish the possible nursing diagnosis as valid or eliminate it as invalid for a particular patient. For example:

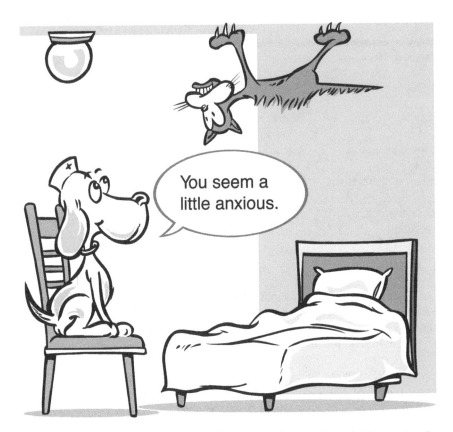

You seem a
little anxious.

FIGURE 3-1.   Both verbal and nonverbal behavior can be used to make the nursing diagnosis of Anxiety.

While caring for a postpartum patient who has delivered a baby born with a cleft lip a few hours before, the nurse anticipates a possible nursing diagnosis of dysfunctional grieving. The nurse hypothesizes that the patient may be feeling guilty, be crying, be angry and sad. The nurse enters the patient's room and, after introducing herself, observes the new mother holding the infant and visually and tactilely exploring the infant's body. The mother speaks gently and warmly to the infant. The nurse asks the patient, "How are you doing with your daughter?" The patient replies, "Well, for a brief moment I was upset with the cleft, but I think my doctor was more upset than I was! You see, I am a nurse also. I work with a plastic surgeon, and I have seen literally hundreds of these conditions. This is nothing! In a couple of months this will be repaired, and it will be impossible to see that anything was wrong. I really trust the surgeon I work for. I can handle this. What if it had been something serious?" At this point the nurse can rule out the possible nursing diagnosis based on the data: maternal bonding, verbal statements of the mother, tactile exploration of the baby's body, nonverbal language of the mother.

COLLABORATIVE PROBLEMS. Some nurses also distinguish between nursing diagnoses that the nurse treats independently and those that the nurse treats collaboratively (jointly shared) with the physician. Nursing and medicine are complementary to each other. Physicians rely on nurses to understand and assess for physiological complications related to patients' medical treatments such as postsurgical phlebitis. The nurse and the physician discuss the problem, and the physician will order new treatments, medications, or intensive monitoring. The nurse carries out these medical orders and continues assessment that is reported to the physician. These types of problems are collaborative. The nurse in this situation is not licensed to prescribe the primary treatment needed to resolve the problem. Much of the assessment and treatment of the problem is directed by the physician even though the nurse may carry it out and adapt it to the particular patient situation. This is interdependent nursing practice. A large part of nursing care involves this kind of collaborative assessment and intervention. In contrast, the independent role of the nurse deals with how the patient responds to actual or at-risk health problems. The nurse not only monitors the patient for these problems but is licensed to diagnose, prescribe, and carry out treatment for these problems. This text considers both independent and interdependent components of nursing practice.

Many nursing diagnoses have both an independent aspect and a collaborative component. For example, there are many measures the nurse may independently use to assist a patient in pain (massage, guided imagery, relaxation techniques), although it is usually a physician's prerogative to order a medication. (Some states give nurse practitioners this practice privilege.) This is an example of a collaborative problem that incorporates independent nursing functions. Other collaborative problems are primarily within the realm of medicine, and the nurse monitors the patient and reports to the physician for medical diagnoses and treatment. Fluid volume deficit is such a collaborative problem. Even though this is a NANDA-approved nursing diagnosis, much of the treatment is determined by the physician and implemented by the nurse. The physician orders the IV and electrolyte replacement, diet therapy, and activity levels, but the nurse is responsible for the implementation. Much of the work of staff nurses in hospitals involves a collaborative role not only with physicians but with professionals in many other disciplines. Nurses share a collaborative role with therapeutic dietitians to resolve the nutritional problems of patients. Psychiatric nurses identify collaborative problems with dance therapists, music therapists, and occupational therapists. The collaborative role is not unique to the disciplines of nursing and medicine.

In addition to deciding if the focus area represents a problem for the patient, the nurse considers a second criterion: Does the problem require nursing intervention to be resolved, lessened, or accommodated? The nurse may identify problems that are clearly within the realm of another health professional. In such a case, the nurse communicates the data to that professional and does not make a diagnosis. This referral to other professionals results in their doing their own assessment and developing a plan to resolve the problem. Nurses may then collaborate in the implementation of the plan as appropriate.

Writing Nursing Diagnoses

ACTUAL NURSING DIAGNOSES. The following formula will result in a clear, concise statement of an *actual (or present) nursing diagnosis*:

Actual Nursing Diagnosis	= Patient Problem + Causes If Known

When writing the diagnosis, the nurse usually replaces the plus symbol with the words "related to," which are abbreviated "r/t." The following are examples of nursing diagnoses in this format:

Actual Nursing Diagnoses

Problem	+	Cause
1. Impaired skin integrity	r/t	Physical immobilization, low oxygen saturation, incontinence
2. Parental role conflict	r/t	Divorce, poor communication
3. Impaired verbal communication	r/t	Inability to speak dominant language

This is a very clear and concise way of writing nursing diagnoses. This is the way nursing diagnoses usually are written in the hospital. The nurse may not always know the cause of the problem and in such a case may simply write "cause unknown."

PES Format. There is another format used for writing actual nursing diagnoses that may be especially helpful for beginning nursing students. Using this approach, which is referred to as PES (Carpenito, 1997), the formula for a nursing diagnosis would look like this:

PES APPROACH

Nursing Diagnosis	=	P Problem	+	E Etiology	+	S Signs and Symptoms

Using this formula, the nurse first selects the approved NANDA nursing diagnosis and then relates it to the cause, which is the same as the etiology. The

signs and symptoms describe the problem, not the etiology. NANDA (1999) suggests signs and symptoms associated with specific nursing diagnoses under the headings "Defining Characteristics" (See Pocket Book). Demonstrating the presence of defining characteristics greatly increases the accuracy of the nursing diagnosis. This may be very helpful to a beginning student, although practicing professional nurses do not often use this longer format. The following would be examples of the same actual nursing diagnoses listed earlier written in the PES format:

1. Impaired skin integrity related to physical immobilization, low oxygen saturation, and incontinence as manifested by disruption of the skin surface over the elbows and coccyx.
2. Parental role conflict related to divorce or poor communication between parents, as manifested by statements of unsatisfactory child care during working hours.
3. Impaired verbal communication related to cultural differences as manifested by inability to speak English.

AT-RISK/HIGH-RISK NURSING DIAGNOSES. For a *high-risk or at-risk nursing diagnosis* the nurse uses the following format:

> At-Risk/High-Risk Nursing Diagnosis = Problem + Risk Factors

When making an at-risk nursing diagnosis, the nurse is unable to list the signs and symptoms because the problem has not yet developed; in fact, the nurse will attempt to intervene so that the problem does not occur. Here the nurse lists the risk factors that have been identified from the assessment that indicate that the problem is very likely to occur. The following are examples of at-risk and high-risk nursing diagnoses:

At-Risk/High-Risk Nursing Diagnoses		
Problem	*+*	*Risk Factor*
1. Risk for impaired skin integrity	r/t	Physical immobilization in total body cast, diaphoresis
2. At risk for fluid volume deficit	r/t	Diarrhea, age 3 yrs, low oral intake, elevated temperature
3. Risk for injury	r/t	Disorientation and decreased vision after (cataract) surgery

POSSIBLE NURSING DIAGNOSES. The nurse may write a *possible nursing diagnosis* as an incomplete problem statement since the validity of the problem is

uncertain but is considered a possibility based on the way many patients respond to similar situations or conditions. Because the purpose of this diagnosis is to assure continued data collection, it is not possible at this stage to identify either signs and symptoms or risk factors. The nurse would merely state the following:

> Possible sensory-perceptual alteration
> Possible nutritional deficit
> Possible fluid volume deficit

Each of these diagnoses requires that the nurse continue to collect sufficient data to make a decision regarding the existence of a nursing problem in this area.

The nurse is now ready to begin writing nursing diagnoses. The following steps summarize the process:

1. Analyze the assessment data.
2. Identify the problem focus area.
3. Consult the NANDA listing of nursing diagnoses to aid in stating the problem. Match the patient's signs and symptoms with the defining characteristics of diagnoses in the problem focus area. Select the diagnosis with the best match.
4. State the cause if known. List as many causes of the problem as possible, since this will be helpful when choosing nursing interventions. For example, if pain is caused by the surgical wound and by movement, interventions can focus on promoting wound healing and giving pain medicines before moving in addition to direct pain management such as analgesics every few hours around the clock.
5. State the signs, symptoms, and risk factors if appropriate.

Occasionally the student will describe a problem that is not included in the NANDA listing. This may reflect an accurate problem. Nursing is an evolving science, and the listing of nursing diagnoses is in the process of development. When this happens, the nurse states the problem as clearly and concisely as possible in a way that communicates the problem to those involved in the care of the patient. The nurse may wish to inform NANDA of this finding and follow the procedure for submitting a new diagnosis for approval and clinical testing. E-mail NANDA@nursecominc.com to share your comments and ideas.

Validating Nursing Diagnoses

When the nurse has completed writing the nursing diagnoses, the ANA *Standards of Clinical Nursing Practice* require that they be validated with the patient, family, and other health care providers when possible and appropriate. This need not be a formal or lengthy session, but the nurse must assure that it occurs. For example, the nurse might bring the care plan to the patient and say, "Mrs. Jones, I have identified some health care problems that I will be using to

plan nursing care during your hospitalization. Could you please help me by telling me if you agree with what I have identified or if I have perhaps missed some that are important to you." This offers patients the opportunity to partici-pate in and make decisions about their care.

CRITICAL THINKING FOR DIAGNOSIS

The activities of data analysis, problem identification, and formulation of the nursing diagnosis all involve critical thinking. The nurse gives meaning to the data on the basis of knowledge and experience and the disciplined completion of the activities in the assessment and diagnosing phases of the nursing process. A critical thinker does not skip steps or base clinical judgments on inadequate data. That type of clinical behavior leads to incorrect diagnoses and errors of omis-sion. One piece of data about voiding difficulty does not lead the nurse to make a nursing diagnosis of *Altered Urinary Elimination*. A critical thinker is still in the "consider this, consider that" stage until more complete data are available. Data may be clustered and reclustered until patterns are recognized. When pat-terns are recognized, more focused data may need to be collected to find addi-tional signs and symptoms to make the diagnosis more certain. The additional data will be used to rule in or rule out the multiple competing nursing diagnoses associated with urinary elimination, for example. A critical thinker also will find out whether the patient interprets the data as a problem before diagnosing the data as a problem.

The nurse will try to identify the etiology of the identified nursing diagno-sis, and again, this involves critical thinking. What are all the possible causes of and contributing factors to this urinary problem? The nurse uses knowledge of the sciences, nursing, and medicine combined with clinical experience, logic, and information about cause and effect and probability to identify the etiology of nursing diagnoses. Critical-thinking skills involve finding patterns in the data and looking for any missing pieces. The nurse considers multiple etiologies for the problem, not just the most obvious one. The nurse and the patient can then discuss these contributing factors and possible ways of eliminating them.

Prompts for Critical Thinking during Diagnosis

- What do the data mean? How do you know? What else could the data mean?
- Are your assessment data accurate? Complete? Are you sure?
- How are these data similar, and how are they different? How are you clus-tering them?
- What assumptions or biases do you have in this situation? Do you think it affected your interpretation of the data or even the data you collected?
- Is your diagnosis supported by enough data?
- Are your statements of etiology (cause of problem) supported by enough data?

- Does the patient see this as a problem? The family? Other health care providers?
- Is this a nursing problem or a collaborative problem? Should you talk to other nurses about this problem or speak with the doctor?
- Have you missed any other problem because you focused only on the obvious one?
- Did you include patient and family strengths, resources, and deficits in your thinking?

CULTURALLY COMPETENT NURSING CARE DURING DIAGNOSIS

Culturally competent care improves the accuracy of nursing diagnoses because the diagnoses are based on a more complete assessment, including consideration of the patient's culture. Health may be viewed as the ability to do work and carry out roles and responsibilities. Physical problems may be secondary and unimportant if one can continue to function in culturally defined ways. In other cultures, the physical problem is the primary focus, not roles and work. This will affect the nursing diagnosis chosen. What do patients view as problems within the context of their culture?

Cultural beliefs and values may be contributing factors for some nursing diagnoses or may be strengths to build on in developing a plan of care. Some examples of nursing diagnoses with cultural contributing factors (etiologies) include the following:

- Impaired verbal communication and inability to speak dominant language related to cultural differences
- Impaired social interaction related to sociocultural conflict, communication barriers, and absence of peers from own culture
- Social isolation related to behavior and values unacceptable to dominant cultural group
- Spiritual distress related to separation from religious and cultural ties and conflict between traditional belief system and Western medical management of disease
- Noncompliance related to conflict between Western medicine and cultural values, beliefs, and health practices.

Prompts for Culturally Competent Nursing Care during Diagnosis

- Does the data base include cultural information from *this* patient?
- Could cultural practices or beliefs be contributing to or causing the current

problem (e.g., diet and obesity; poor fluid intake and inappropriate temperature of fluids at bedside)?

- Are the nursing diagnoses you select interpreted as "problems" by patients from different cultures or only in the Western medical culture?
- Does the patient or family believe something is a problem from their cultural perspective that the nurse does not view as a problem from the Western medical perspective?
- Is the physical problem the correct nursing diagnosis, or is the problem interference with roles and responsibilities caused by the physical problem?

DIAGNOSIS

Turning a Negative into a Positive

As part of developing a nursing diagnosis, careful analysis of the facts and accurate problem identification are needed. The more obvious nursing diagnosis of dysfunctional grieving *was almost made for a patient with a truly different problem. The nurse manager of the vascular unit had a Native American shaman (medicine man) in her office who was requesting retrieval of a tribe member's limb after amputation. We had never had such a request, and the operating room was unsure how to proceed. In speaking with the shaman, I learned that it was important to this tribe that when death occurred, the person be buried whole. This practice allowed the totality of the spirit to advance after death. The patient and family were already grieving for the loss of the limb. Added to this situation would have been* spiritual distress *about the inability of the body and spirit to reunite as a whole after death.*

How were we going to honor the shaman's request of allowing the limb to leave the hospital and maintain our hospital practice of not giving out such items after surgery? The problem was how to transport the limb out of the hospital without violating infection control. After further discussion and some research, the shaman was able to remove the limb properly cleansed and wrapped. This allowed the patient and his family to conclude the hospitalization with a tribal passing ritual and properly bury the limb. If one properly analyzes the facts of a situation and then looks openly at persons' wishes, a nursing diagnosis can be made that positively influences the patient's outcome.

R. Peterson, RN, MSN

FIGURE 3-2.

NURSING DIAGNOSIS: THE MANAGED CARE ENVIRONMENT

Patients receiving care in all settings of the health care continuum are faced with the high cost of care. Payers of ambulatory surgery, outpatient clinic care, inpatient hospital care, and home health care all require some justification that the care was medically necessary and appropriate. Payers most often rely on communication from registered nurses on the hospital staff to receive clinical information. The nurses charged with this responsibility are usually case managers or members of an institution's utilization review department. These nurses rely on the medical record as an important source of the clinical information relayed to payers. Both physicians and staff nurses caring for patients have an obligation to document clinical data that will assure that the patient's condition is represented accurately in the medical record. This is one way to help patients obtain the insurance coverage to which they are entitled. The documentation should not be overstated or understated. It should describe the condition of the patient accurately and factually.

Documentation of the patient's condition can be done in several ways: an admission note, placement of the patient on a critical pathway, or adding to a multidisciplinary problem list. Upon completing an admission nursing assessment and identifying nursing diagnoses, the staff nurse completes an admission note. This notation in the medical record describes the patient's condition and the reason the patient gave for seeking health care. Often nurses choose to write this as a direct quote. For example, a nurse who is admitting a patient complaining of chest pain may write: "Patient states: 'The pain was so bad, I thought I was going to die.'"

Another way to document the patient's condition is by selecting a critical pathway that reflects the patient's condition or surgical procedure. The staff nurse selects a critical pathway related to a particular medical diagnosis and DRG and reviews it for appropriateness for the individual patient. The nursing diagnoses identified in the pathway have been established by expert nurses and have been found to be valid for the vast majority of patients with a particular medical diagnosis. The admission note that the nurse makes includes documentation about the choice of pathway, for example, "Patient placed on total knee replacement critical pathway." Some insurance companies choose to review the critical pathways an institution has developed. If the insurance company agrees with the reasonableness of the care as delineated in the pathway, it often does not require further information from the care providers unless the patient's condition requires a longer stay or significant changes from the pathway. Some institutions have developed critical pathways that are begun in the clinic and move the patient through hospital admission and home care. The requirements of patient assessment, identification of additional individualized nursing diagnoses, and review of the pathway for this unique patient are the same in all settings.

It is also important that the nurse evaluate and document the severity of the patient's illness. One clue in thinking about this is to consider the following: What is there about this patient's need that requires the care to be given in this setting? For example, a patient is admitted to the hospital with severe chest pain. She has had prior episodes of chest pain that were relieved by nitroglycerin. On this admission, blood pressure (BP) is 108/60, pain is 7 on a 10-point scale and is not relieved by nitroglycerin, and the patient complains of being unable to breathe because of the "crushing pain." The nurse documents a nursing history and assessment and begins to consider possible nursing diagnoses: acute pain, ineffective breathing pattern, altered cardiopulmonary tissue perfusion, inability to maintain spontaneous ventilation. This patient will require skilled assessment and intensive monitoring by registered nurses. The requirement of intensive monitoring and assessment is the most common reason why patients need to be admitted to the hospital. If this requirement is not present, it may be the patient could be cared for in a less expensive setting, perhaps with home care or at a skilled nursing facility.

Another way to describe the patient's condition is through the use of a multidisciplinary problem list. This method is most often used in the ambulatory setting. The list includes a dated statement of the problem that is given a number, the signature and discipline of the staff member originating the problem, and a blank for the date of resolution of the problem and the signature of the person evaluating the problem. In all the documentation that follows, the staff members use the number of the problem to refer back to the problem list. The problem list is usually the first document in the ambulatory or clinic medical record. The following is an example of a problem list for a 17-year-old female seen by a nurse practitioner for primary care. Note that the list is ongoing and in reverse chronological order so that it is added to at each visit.

Ms. Jennifer Smith   Date of birth: 6/2/1983

	Problem	Date	Discipline	Signature	Resolution
1.	Painful menstruation	10/96	Medicine		
2.	Otitis media (swimmer's ear)	6/97	Medicine		
3.	Alteration in nutrition: more than body requirements	9/99	Nursing		
4.	Situational depression	11/99	Psychiatric consult		

Any method of documentation that is consistent with institutional policy is acceptable as long as the patient's condition is clearly reflected. Remember that the documentation must accurately reflect the severity of illness of the patient.

SUMMARY

The process of diagnosing consists of three activities: data analysis, problem identification, and the formulation of nursing diagnoses. During data analysis the nurse makes decisions based on the data regarding the health status of the patient. Next the nurse identifies problem focus areas, and finally the nurse states a nursing diagnosis. The nursing diagnosis includes the patient problem and its cause or etiology if known. The statement may also include signs and symptoms *if* the student is using the PES format. If the patient is at risk for developing a certain problem, the nurse makes an at-risk or high-risk nursing diagnosis and includes the identification of the risk factors that determined the diagnosis.

PRACTICE EXERCISE

Pick out the correctly written nursing diagnoses. Identify what is wrong with the incorrectly written nursing diagnoses. (Either the abbreviated formula or the PES formula is acceptable.) The correct answers follow the exercise.

1. Alteration in nutrition: less than body requirements related to nausea after chemotherapy.
2. Range of motion exercises (ROM) after a cerebral vascular accident (CVA).
3. Cancer of the breast with metastasis to the axillary lymph nodes.
4. Refusing wound irrigation related to pain of procedure.
5. Body image disturbance related to amputation of right foot.
6. Risk for sexual dysfunction in relating to husband and friends related to mastectomy.
7. Intermittent positive pressure breathing (IPPB) exercises qid to increase lung expansion
8. Pain and fear related to surgical procedure.
9. Severe itching related to a fungal infection.
10. Activity intolerance related to shortness of breath on activity.
11. Impaired physical mobility associated with right-sided paralysis.
12. Ineffective breathing pattern, etiology unknown, as evidenced by shortness of breath, tachypnea, pursed-lip breathing.
13. Disorientation to time and place related to confused state.
14. Impaired verbal communication related to inability to speak dominant English language.

15. Fear related to uncertain outcome of surgery as manifested by urinary frequency, irritability, rapid pulse, "It's all I can think about—I'm sure it's cancer."
16. Ambulate progressively with tripod cane.
17. Risk for infection related to second-degree burns on right hand.
18. Patient is upset and worried about the cost of hospitalization.
19. Impaired skin integrity related to prolonged bed rest as manifested by skin breakdown over both elbows and coccyx.
20. Thrombophlebitis related to prolonged bed rest as manifested by a positive Homan's sign.

ANSWERS TO EXERCISE ON NURSING DIAGNOSIS

1. Correct. Problem = less than body requirements for nutritional needs,
            Cause   = nausea after chemotherapy
   In this case nursing care will focus on methods to relieve the nausea.
2. Incorrect.
   Range of motion exercises are a nursing intervention.
3. Incorrect.
   Cancer of the breast is a medical diagnosis, one which the nurse is not licensed to treat. An experienced nurse might anticipate possible nursing diagnoses having to do with pain, body image, fear, or anxiety.
4. Incorrect.
   This is a nursing problem. The real nursing diagnosis may be something like Pain associated with irrigation procedure. There would be many things the nurse could do to deal with the pain and make the procedure more acceptable to the patient.
5. Correct. Problem = body image disturbance
            Cause   = amputation of the right foot
6. Correct. Problem = risk for sexual dysfunction
            Cause   = related to mastectomy
7. Incorrect. This is a medical treatment.
8. Incorrect. These are two separate problems that will each require different nursing care.
9. Correct. Problem = severe itching
            Cause   = fungal infection
   While this diagnosis is not listed in a NANDA format, it does clearly convey the patient problem. However, the nurse does need additional information regarding the location of the infection. In this case the PES format would be helpful. The signs and symptoms might include patient complaints, scratch marks and rash on right leg, restlessness.
10. Incorrect. SOB is not a cause but a sign/symptom. Need etiology if known in diagnostic statement.

11. Correct.
12. Correct. P = ineffective breathing pattern
    E = unknown
    S = shortness of breath, tachypnea, pursed-lip breathing
13. Incorrect. Problem and cause are the same.
14. Correct. Problem = impaired verbal communication
    Cause   = inability to speak dominant English language
15. Correct. P = Fear
    E = uncertain outcome of surgery
    S = urinary frequency, irritability, rapid pulse, "It's all I can
    think about—I'm sure it's cancer."
16. Incorrect. This is a physician's order.
17. Correct. Problem = risk for infection
    Cause   = related to second-degree burns on right hand
18. Incorrect. This is a judgment. It may indicate that there is a problem, but
    additional data are needed. This may be a problem that the nurse will refer
    to a social worker who has additional resources to assist this patient.
19. Correct. P = impaired skin integrity
    E = related to prolonged bed rest
    S = skin breakdown over coccyx and both elbows
20. Incorrect. This is a medical diagnosis, but it would suggest possible nurs-
    ing diagnoses related to physical safety and pain. These diagnoses would
    need further patient data for confirmation.

CASE STUDY: NURSING DIAGNOSES

The case study of Mrs. Wiley is continued from Chapter 2 to identify nursing diagnoses. The NANDA-approved diagnostic categories are used. Two different formats are used to state the diagnosis of an actual problem. The first format uses the three parts: problem identification, etiology, and signs and symptoms of the problem (PES format). The second format uses two parts: problem identification and etiology. The signs and symptoms are listed under the category "supporting data." Note that the nursing diagnosis of *knowledge deficit* requires that the nurse specify the particular knowledge or skill the patient lacks. The two-part format is not used for *knowledge deficit*.

NURSING DIAGNOSIS #1

Preoperative Orthopedic Surgery Clinic

Mrs. Wiley: Nursing diagnoses identified by the nurse in the orthopedic clinic.

Example 1:

   a. Knowledge deficit: strengthening exercises, crutch walking, pain management after surgery (PCA), use of incentive spirometer, preoperative preparation for surgery as evidenced by patient statement that she has never been hospitalized and does not know what to expect. (PES format)

   b. Knowledge deficit: strengthening exercises, crutch walking, pain management after surgery, use of incentive spirometer, preoperative preparation for surgery.

      Supporting data: "I have never been hospitalized except for a maternity stay—no idea what to expect."

Example 2:

   a. Husband: risk for injury related to absence of care provider as evidenced by patient statement that she cares for her frail, elderly husband and is concerned that "he is not safe overnight alone." (PES format)

   b. Husband: risk for injury related to absence of care provider.

      Supporting data: lives with 80-year-old husband, who is frail and weak. "I don't know what he would do without me. He can't cook for himself or really be safe overnight alone. What if he fell?"

Example 3:

   a. Chronic pain related to degeneration of knee joint as evidenced by patient statement: "I need to have my knee joint replaced. I have been trying to avoid it, but now the pain is too much." (PES format)

   b. Chronic pain related to degeneration of knee joint.

      Supporting data: patient statement: "I need to have my knee joint replaced. I have been trying to avoid it, but now the pain is too much. I try to stay off it as much as possible, but I like to play golf and really cannot do that because of the pain. I take Motrin or Tylenol for the pain, but lately that doesn't help."

NURSING DIAGNOSIS #2

First Day Surgery Center: 6 A.M.

Patients are admitted to the first day surgery center the morning of surgery for their scheduled procedures and are transferred to the inpatient unit after surgery.

Mrs. Wiley: Nursing diagnoses identified by the nurse at the time of admission, 6 A.M. on the day of surgery.

Example 1

a. Fear of reduced mobility related to outcome of surgery as evidenced by patient statement: "What if the surgery makes it worse?" (PES format)

b. Fear of reduced mobility related to outcome of surgery.

Supporting data: Patient statement: "What if the surgery makes it worse?"

Example 2:

a. Risk for injury (Mrs. Wiley) related to inexperienced crutch walking as evidenced by patient statement: "I have practiced crutch walking but don't feel comfortable with it yet" and physical therapist's note that patient needs additional instructions after surgery and a walker. (PES format)

b. Risk for injury (Mrs. Wiley) related to inexperienced crutch walking.

Supporting data: patient statement: "I have practiced crutch walking but don't feel comfortable with it yet" and physical therapist's note that patient needs additional instructions after surgery and a walker.

Example 3:

a. Anxiety (patient/family) related to surgical experience and unfamiliar environment as evidenced by shakiness, jitters (Mrs. W.), trembling voice (daughter and husband), darting eye movements (husband); patient has not been in hospital. (PES format)

b. Anxiety (patient/family) related to surgical experience and unfamiliar environment.

Supporting data: shakiness, jitters (Mrs. W.), trembling voice (daughter and husband), darting eye movements (husband); patient has not been in hospital.

NURSING DIAGNOSIS #3

Postoperative Orthopedic Patient Care Unit

Mrs. Wiley: Nursing diagnoses identified by the nurses on the inpatient nursing unit.

Example 1:

a. Acute pain related to joint replacement surgery, physical therapy, movement as evidenced by pain rating (6–8), restlessness, change in vital signs: increased pulse, respirations, and BP. (PES format)

b. Acute pain related to joint replacement surgery, physical therapy, and movement.

Supporting data: patient pain rating (6–8), restlessness, change in vital signs: increased pulse, respirations, and BP.

Example 2:

a. Risk for caregiver role strain (upon discharge) related to dependency of frail spouse and surgery of caregiver as evidenced by husband statements, his inability to eat/sleep, Mrs. Wiley's concerns about his safety when she is not home. (PES format)

b. Risk for caregiver role strain (upon discharge) related to dependency of frail spouse and surgery of caregiver.

Supporting data: husband statements, his inability to eat/sleep, Mrs. Wiley's concerns about his safety when she is not home.

Example 3:

a. Impaired physical mobility, level 2 (requires help from another person for assistance, supervision, and teaching), related to knee replacement surgery as evidenced by pain, need for assistance with turning, repositioning, weakness, and fatigue. (PES format)

b. Impaired physical mobility, level 2, related to knee replacement surgery.

Supporting data: pain, need for assistance with turning, repositioning, weakness, and fatigue.

Example 4: Nurse continues this diagnosis from preoperative plan.

a. Risk for injury (Mrs. Wiley) related to inexperienced crutch walking as evidenced by patient statement: "I have practiced crutch walking but don't feel comfortable with it yet" and physical therapist's note that patient needs additional instructions after surgery and probably a walker. (PES format)

b. Risk for injury (Mrs. Wiley) related to inexperienced crutch walking.

Supporting data: patient statement: "I have practiced crutch walking but don't feel comfortable with it yet" and physical therapist's note that patient needs additional instructions after surgery and probably a walker.

NURSING DIAGNOSIS #4

Home Health Care Agency

Mrs. Wiley: These nursing diagnoses were identified by the registered nurse at the time of the first home visit.

Example 1:

   a. Knowledge/skill deficit: signs/symptoms to report to MD; aseptic technique; self-administered medication, purpose, schedule; wound care; pain management techniques as evidenced by patient statement: "They really talked about all that while I was in the hospital, but I was just too scared to absorb it. I can't remember what I am supposed to do when—or even how to do it." (PES format)

   b. Knowledge/skill deficit: signs/symptoms to report to MD; aseptic technique; self-administered medication, purpose, schedule; wound care; pain management techniques.

       Supporting data: "They really talked about all that while I was in the hospital, but I was just too scared to absorb it. I can't remember what I am supposed to do when—or even how to do it."

Example 2:

   a. Acute pain related to joint replacement surgery, physical therapy, and movements as evidenced by pain rating 3–4 and patient statement: "It is less painful if I just stay put and do not move." (PES format)

   b. Acute pain related to joint replacement surgery, physical therapy, and movement.

       Supporting data: pain rating of 3–4 and patient statement: "It is less painful if I just stay put and do not move."

Example 3:

   a. Risk for injury (Mrs. Wiley) related to inexperienced crutch walking as evidenced by patient statement: "I was in too much pain in the hospital to really work at it. It is one thing to do it with the therapist in the hospital, but my home is carpeted and a lot trickier. I really feel safer with a walker." (PES format)

b. Risk for injury (Mrs. Wiley) related to inexperienced crutch walking.

Supporting data: patient statement: "I was in too much pain in the hospital to really work at it. It is one thing to do it with the therapist in the hospital, but my home is carpeted and a lot trickier. I really feel safer with a walker."

CHAPTER 4

Outcome Identification

STANDARD III. OUTCOME IDENTIFICATION

The Nurse Identifies Expected Outcomes Individualized to the Patient.

Reprinted with permission from American Nurses Association, *Standards of Clinical Nursing Practice*, 2nd edition, © 1998 American Nurses Publishing, American Nurses Foundation/American Nurses Association, Washington, D.C.

Now that the nurse has collected data about a patient, analyzed the data, and formulated some nursing diagnoses, the outcome identification phase of the nursing process begins. In this phase, the nurse develops outcomes for the patient to achieve showing an optimum or improved level of functioning in the problem areas identified in the nursing diagnoses. The nurse analyzes the strengths and weaknesses of the patient, the patient's family, the nursing personnel, the health care facility, and the available resources (including other health care professionals). The nurse also examines personal strengths, beliefs, and values that might affect outcome identification. A nurse who is unable or unwilling to work with a patient in a particular problem area may need to seek help from another, more experienced staff nurse, clinical instructor, or other resource.

Outcomes are developed to make nursing care both individualized for the patient and realistic for the hospital or home care setting. The skills of problem solving and decision making are applied to a particular patient's identified problems. The resulting outcomes and plan of nursing care are designed to help patients and their families
—make informed decisions about their health and health care
—maintain their current level of health and functioning if they are identified as being at risk for developing problems
—avoid injury or disease
—regain a previous level of health and functioning
—reach an improved level of health and functioning
—adjust to a reduced level of health and functioning when improvement is not possible
—adapt to a progressively decreasing level of functioning
—experience a peaceful death

ACTIVITIES IN THE OUTCOME IDENTIFICATION PHASE

There are two steps in the outcome identification phase: setting priorities among the nursing diagnoses when a patient has several problems and establishing outcomes with a patient and family to help lessen or eliminate the health problems.

$$\frac{\text{Outcome}}{\text{Identification}} = \frac{\text{Setting}}{\text{Priorities}} + \frac{\text{Establishing}}{\text{Outcomes}}$$

SETTING PRIORITIES

During the process of priority setting, the nurse and the patient, whenever possible, mutually determine which problems identified during the diagnosis phase are in need of immediate attention and which problems may be dealt with later. Consider assigning identified patient problems a high, middle, or low priority. The higher-priority problems deserve the most immediate nursing attention for a plan and treatment. Setting priorities serves the purpose of ordering the delivery of nursing care so that more important or life threatening problems are treated before less critical problems are treated. Priority setting does not mean that one problem must be totally resolved before another problem is considered. Problems frequently can be approached simultaneously. At times, decreasing the severity of one problem works to eliminate the others, as occurs when eliminating severe pain corrects an ineffective breathing pattern.

Guidelines for Setting Priorities

1. Maslow's hierarchy of basic needs can guide the selection of high-priority problems. Survival needs that are significantly unmet pose the greatest threat to life and functioning and thus deserve a high-priority rating. Using Maslow's theory to guide the delivery of nursing care, the nurse would do the following:
   —Relieve a patient's pain (physiological need) before encouraging morning hygiene (self-esteem)
   —Encourage a new mother to express her disappointment about having a C-section when she had planned on totally natural childbirth (self-esteem) before teaching her infant-care skills (self-actualization)
   —Stabilize bleeding and ensure adequate oxygenation in an emergency room accident victim before assessing elimination status (both of these

are basic physiological needs, but oxygenation is usually the highest-priority need; bleeding is considered a threat to tissue oxygenation)
—Consider how difficult it is for you to read and absorb the material in this book (self-actualization need) if you have had too little sleep (physiological need)

Basic survival needs usually take priority over higher level needs if the survival needs are not being satisfied. This is the case when a patient is in obvious physical distress owing to the unmet need. If the survival needs are being partially met and actual physical distress is tolerable, a higher level need may take priority over or at least have the same priority as a lower level need. For example, an auto accident victim can be in considerable distress with multiple physical needs unmet, yet the priority need may be to ascertain the whereabouts and injuries of the other family members in the car when it crashed. This unmet higher level need can have a negative effect on satisfaction of this patient's physical needs if it is not given appropriate attention.

2. Focus on the problems the patient feels are most important if this priority does not interfere with medical treatment. A patient's need for undisturbed rest cannot take precedence over a medically ordered treatment for observation of blood pressure and pulse every hour after a car accident.

If there are no nursing contraindications, offer patients the opportunity to set their own priorities. However, do not offer them the opportunity to make choices they really do not have or are not qualified to make. After surgery, the patient and family may identify the need for rest and pain management as priority concerns, while the nurse is equally concerned about maintaining a clear airway and improving gas exchange based on an assessment of diminished breath sounds and moist gurgling heard in the lungs. The challenge for the nurse is to help all the involved parties understand and agree about which problems will be dealt with now and which may have to wait until the patient is more stable.

Mutual priority setting with the patient serves two purposes. First, this approach involves patients in planning their own care. Perhaps the nurse has overlooked a major problem that is consuming the patient's time and energy or has assigned the problem a low priority. Unless this problem is considered first, the nurse may be able to achieve only limited success in other areas because the patient is still worrying about the overlooked problem. Second, cooperation between the nurse and the patient is enhanced when priority setting is done together. The nurse often acts as a negotiator by stating recognition of patient and family concerns, sharing nursing and medical concerns with them, and guiding priority setting to promote safe physical care. The nurse also identifies patient/family concerns to the physician, other nurses, and other health care professionals, who may then reset their priorities based on a better understanding of the patient's status.

3. Consider the patient's culture, values, and beliefs when setting priorities. Nurses are increasingly working with patients and families from cultures other than the dominant culture in which most nurses grew up and were edu-

cated. Patients may hold very different views of health and health care, and those beliefs cannot be ignored. Instead, they should be respected and considered in priority setting whenever possible.

4. Consider the effect of potential problems when setting priorities. For example:
   — A new mother may ask to be left alone with her husband and newborn to get acquainted. The potential collaborative problem of a postpartum hemorrhage developing would require continuous observation after delivery, since this is potentially life threatening. Thus, the patient's request to be left alone cannot be safely met.
   — A bedridden patient may be started on a routine of frequent turning and positioning to prevent bed sores and contractures even though the patient may not see this as important. Prevention of the potential complications associated with prolonged bed rest is a high priority, since treating these problems after they develop is less effective, more costly, and usually more time-consuming than preventive measures.

   Prevention of a high-risk problem, rather than treatment of the problem when it develops, is an outcome that deserves continuous assessment and intervention.

5. Consider costs, resources available, personnel, and time needed to plan for and treat each of the patient's identified problems. If resources, personnel time or financing are currently unavailable to deal with a particular problem, it may receive a low priority until some of these obstacles have been overcome. If a problem can be resolved quickly, it may receive a high priority for practical reasons.

6. Consider state laws, hospital policy statements, and outcome criteria established for the particular setting. For example, in many states it is the law that all children under age 4 years be transported in an approved car seat. Hospital policy may state that newborns must be taken home by their parents in an appropriate car seat. This potential problem of injury to a newborn who is not in a car seat during an automobile accident should be discussed early to give the family time to obtain a car seat before discharge.

ESTABLISHING OUTCOMES

After setting priorities, the nurse will establish outcomes for each of the patient's problems identified by the nursing diagnoses. An outcome is a "measurable, expected, client-focused goal" (ANA, 1998) to be achieved at some specified time in the future. For an *actual nursing diagnosis* where the problem currently exists, the outcome describes a future change in the patient's health status or functioning showing a reduction or lessening of the problem. For an *at-risk*

nursing diagnosis that does not currently exist but has a high probability of occurring without preventive nursing interventions, the outcome is often to maintain the current problem-free status or level of functioning.

Patient Outcome

The desired result of nursing care; that which you hope to achieve with your patient and which is designed to prevent, remedy, or lessen the problem identified in the nursing diagnosis.

Why Is an Outcome Statement Needed?

Outcomes are needed as part of the plan of care because they tell the nurse and the patient where they are going. They should be part of the nurse's thinking whenever care is given. "Where am I going with this patient today? Where do we hope to be in relation to lessening or resolving a particular problem by the end of my shift?" The outcomes give guidance in the selection of nursing interventions. Outcomes are constant future targets to remind all caregivers and the patient why certain activities or interventions are done. Outcomes give a standard against which to compare the patient's hourly, daily, weekly, monthly, yearly, and lifelong efforts to maintain and improve health and functioning. Outcomes give a sense of where this particular patient started from and where the individual and the nurse hope to end up. The assessment data provide the *baseline* for the patient's current level of function in a problem area. For example, a newly diagnosed diabetic has lost 20 lbs, is dehydrated, and is inadequately nourished. The outcome might be for the individual to regain 15 lbs over the next 2 months, taking his prescribed amount of insulin each day. Progress toward this outcome over the weeks will be measured against the original baseline data and the optimal weight gain identified in the outcome statement. The outcomes nurses write will be the criteria used to evaluate the success of nursing interventions. An outcome helps motivate the nurse, the patient, and the family to continue their efforts. When outcomes are achieved, it provides everyone involved with the reward of success, and success promotes further efforts to achieve additional, higher level outcomes.

The outcome for a student in nursing might be to graduate from school with a GPA of 3.0. Another student might set higher or lower outcome criteria that depend on competing life responsibilities and personal abilities. The same is true in nursing practice. Without a clear, concise outcome statement, the nurse and the patient do not know if and when the desired end has been achieved.

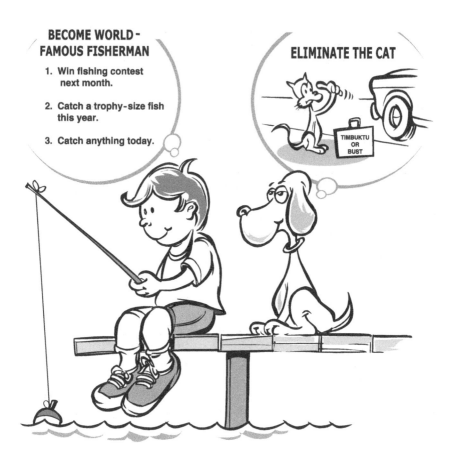

FIGURE 4-1.   Identifying individualized outcomes.

Components of an Outcome Statement

At least one outcome is written for each nursing diagnosis. Generally, several outcomes are written for each diagnosis, especially if there is a broad scope to the problem. Outcomes are written to include specific components that are identified in the box below.

Outcome Statement	=	Patient Behavior	+	Criteria of Performance	+	Conditions (If Needed)	+	Time Frame

PATIENT BEHAVIOR.   The patient behavior the nurse selects for the outcome statement is an observable activity the patient will demonstrate after a series of nursing interventions. The activity is observable in that it can be seen, heard, felt, or measured by the nurse or reported by the patient. The activity chosen

shows an improved level of functioning in the problem area identified in the nursing diagnosis. If the nursing diagnosis is an at-risk problem versus an actual current problem, the activity selected will reflect maintenance of the current status or level of functioning. The activity selected for the outcome should not deal with the etiology of the problem as stated in the nursing diagnosis but should address a lessening or elimination of the problem. For example:

Nursing Diagnosis: Pain related to movement, coughing, and tissue trauma secondary to surgery.

Patient Behavior: "Patient rates pain as a 3 or less . . ." (deals with problem of pain) versus "Patient demonstrates splinting of incision when cough-' ing . . ." (deals with etiology of problem, not directly with the pain).

The etiology of the pain problem above will be dealt with when the nurse selects interventions to meet the outcome of decreased pain. If the patient can meet the outcome as written and still have no reduction in pain, the outcome is incorrectly written. It is probably focused on the etiology part of the nursing diagnosis and is a nursing intervention rather than an outcome. In the example above, teaching the patient to splint and support the incision before turning or coughing is an intervention to help achieve the outcome of having the patient rate the pain at 3 or less.

In writing an outcome statement, the word *client* or *patient* or the actual name of the person may be omitted since the outcome always refers to the patient.

PATIENT BEHAVIOR = an observable activity the patient will demonstrate at some time in the future showing improvement in the problem area

—(the patient) will drink   (for a problem with hydration)
—(the patient) will void   (for an elimination problem)
—decrease in (the patient's) weight   (for a nutrition problem)
—(the patient) will ambulate   (for a mobility problem)
—states steps in self-catheterization   (for a knowledge deficit diagnosis)

A caution is warranted about writing an outcome stating that the patient will attend some type of class or meeting. Answer the question, Why do you want the patient to attend this class or meeting? What outcome do you hope for? Unless the problem is social isolation or loneliness, this type of outcome statement is usually an intervention rather than an outcome. If the diagnosis is a knowledge deficit, attending a class in the area of the deficit is not an outcome. It is an intervention. The patient could attend the class and learn nothing and still meet this type of outcome. The real outcome would be for the patient to state or demonstrate the knowledge or skill the nurse hoped was learned by attending the class.

CRITERION OF PERFORMANCE.   The criterion of performance is a stated level or standard for the patient behavior stated in the outcome. This part of the outcome specifies a realistic improvement in functioning in the problem area by a stated time and will be used to determine whether the outcome was satisfactorily

achieved. The criterion clarifies and individualizes the outcome based on the patient's abilities and a realistic expectation for the level of functioning in the future. If the behavior selected for the outcome is to pass the course Nsg 101, is a grade of "D" an acceptable criterion for achievement or should the minimum criterion be set at the "C" level? Some outcomes identify the optimum level of recovery or functioning for a patient after treatment and nursing care and often span days, weeks, or months. The time frame portion of the outcome statement is addressed further in this section and will affect the criterion selected for each outcome. The level of functioning a patient can achieve this shift or this week may be very different from a long-term total recovery criterion. Consider the time frame when selecting the criterion. The shorter the time frame, the smaller the expected progress toward elimination of the problem.

CRITERION OF ACCEPTABLE PERFORMANCE = the level at which the patient will perform the behavior. How well? How far? How much?
—at least 500 ml of fluids
—250 ml of urine or more
—at least 5 lbs
—the length of the hall and back
—without contamination of the syringe
—accurately and safely

CONDITIONS.   Sometimes the nurse sets outcomes with the patient that require the use or presence of certain environmental conditions. Conditions can be thought of as specific aids that will help the patient perform a behavior at the level specified in the criteria portion of the outcome statement. Not all outcomes will have a condition. If the condition is essential to the performance of the behavior, include it. If it is not essential, leave it out.

CONDITIONS = the circumstances, if necessary, under which the behavior will be performed
—with the use of a walker
—with the use of a wheelchair
—with the help of the family
—with the use of medication
—while on oxygen
—on twice-daily insulin injections
—while on a patient-controlled analgesia (PCA) machine

TIME FRAME.   The outcome statement includes a time or date to clarify how long it would realistically take for the patient to reach the level of functioning stated in the criteria part of the outcome. This is based on nursing knowledge, experience, and knowledge of the individual patient. The time frames stated in the outcome may be minutes, hours, days, weeks, or months. Intermediate outcomes may be achieved relatively sooner compared with long-term outcomes, which usually span the time it would take for most patients to achieve maximum recovery.

a. Intermediate outcomes. Intermediate outcomes identify behavior a patient can achieve fairly quickly, in a matter of hours, in an 8-hour shift, or on a daily basis. Occasionally intermediate outcomes will involve weeks or months in a long-term care facility or in home health nursing, where maximum recovery is expected to take months or years. Intermediate outcomes are especially appropriate to acute care settings, such as hospitals, where most patients stay only a few days and continue to recover at home or in a long-term care facility.

If a problem is diagnosed that tends to worsen with the passage of time, in terms of hours or days, intermediate outcomes are more appropriate than long-term or final outcomes to guide care. The nurse wants to see a change in patient behavior soon; the problem cannot be allowed to continue until physical or psychological damage occurs. For example, a patient who is unable to void after surgery cannot be left for 24 hours with a filling bladder. Extreme discomfort and possible damage to the bladder or kidneys could be the consequence. An intermediate outcome is identified for a patient after surgery, such as "reestablishment of urinary elimination within 6 hours after surgery." If the patient is unable to achieve this intermediate outcome, a catheter is often inserted to empty the bladder and prevent damage. Not all intermediate outcomes are written on a patient's plan of care. Working toward outcomes is a way of thinking. Rather than thinking of separate tasks to accomplish this shift, such as bedbath, VS, ROM exercises, and meds, the nurse thinks, "What can I realistically accomplish with this patient in the next few hours to help lessen or eliminate the diagnosed problem?"

Some examples of intermediate outcomes are the following:

Respirations below 30 breaths/minute within 1 hour.
Return of bowel sounds within 12 hours postop.
Passing flatus within 24 hours postop.
Temperature to be below 102° F within 1 hour.
Pain to be rated as 4 or less within 30 minutes.
For the reader of this book: completion of Chapter 4 in the next hour.

When learning to write outcomes, start with intermediate outcomes. A beginning nursing student is not with the same patient for long periods of time. Students may care for a patient for only a few hours. By writing intermediate outcomes involving the length of time with the patient, the student will be able to give the needed nursing care and evaluate the results. By evaluating whether the intermediate outcome was met before leaving the patient, students will gain skill in writing realistic outcomes and giving nursing care to meet those goals.

Intermediate outcomes often are developed to help the nurse and the patient gauge progress toward final outcomes. By achieving intermediate outcomes, the patient is gradually advanced to the improved or optimum level of functioning identified in the final outcome. Achievement of intermediate outcomes provides repeated satisfaction for both the nurse and the patient, serving as evidence of progress and guidance for the future. For example, the nurse and the patient have

identified an outcome of "weight loss of 80 pounds in 1 year." Progressive intermediate outcomes are identified to help the nurse and the patient measure
progress toward achievement of the eventual outcome. For example:

Weight of 210 pounds by February 7.
Weight of 208 pounds by February 14.
Weight of 206 pounds by February 21.

A series of intermediate outcomes that a person can realistically accomplish
in a stated time period is much more rewarding than is striving for one long-term
outcome. The repeated reinforcement a person receives from meeting intermediate outcomes can keep an individual motivated to achieve a final outcome. If
intermediate outcomes are not achieved, new nursing interventions can be tried,
more realistic outcomes can be selected, or the nurse may reanalyze the data and
diagnosis to make sure the problem is accurately identified and important to the
patient and family.

Some other examples of intermediate outcomes leading to long-term outcomes include the following:

1. "I will finish reading this book before final exams" might be a long-term
   outcome for a student in nursing. This student might accomplish the long-
   term outcome through progressive intermediate outcomes of reading one
   chapter each week.
2. "Patient will demonstrate full use of broken arm within 6 months." This
   patient might accomplish the long-term outcome by progressively increasing the amount and range of muscle/joint exercises.
3. "Performance of self-care activities within 3 months of cerebral vascular
   accident (stroke)." Progressive intermediate outcomes might focus on the
   accomplishment of one self-care activity a week until the patient is able to
   perform all activities independently (final outcome).
   Week of 10/10: Feeds self by end of week.
   Week of 10/17: Brushes teeth by end of week.
   Week of 10/24: Performs personal hygiene by end of week.
   Week of 10/31: Meets own mobility needs by end of week.

b. Long-term or final outcomes. Long-term outcomes give direction for
nursing care over time. These outcomes can be thought of as an eventual destination, whereas progressive intermediate outcomes are a series of stops on the
way to the final destination of optimum recovery. Intermediate and final outcomes are similar to a cross-country car trip. You plan to be in Florida by March
28. To achieve that long-term outcome, you must be in Chicago by March 25
and in Georgia by March 27. These stops along the way are intermediate outcomes to assist the eventual achievement of the long-term outcome. Long-term
outcomes try to identify the maximum level of functioning possible for a patient
with a particular nursing diagnosis. Consider the prognosis of the patient's

health problems, resources available, strengths and weaknesses of the patient and family, and nursing care abilities of the personnel who will be working with the patient. If the patient has an alteration in some function, the long-term outcome is to restore a normal pattern of functioning if possible. If that is not possible, the outcome deals with establishing a maximum level of functioning for the alteration and helping the patient to adjust to this altered level of functioning. Some examples of long-term outcomes include the following:

Reestablishment of patient's usual bowel elimination patterns in 2 months.
Reestablishment of normal voiding patterns by 5 days postop.
Breast-feeding 10 to 15 minutes/breast, every 2 to 5 hours, within 2 weeks of delivery.
Self-care of colostomy 1 month after surgery.
Patient to state no longer afraid of having severe pain during terminal illness from cancer after 1 week on IV morphine pump.
For the reader of this book: utilization of the nursing process to assess, diagnose, identify outcomes, plan, implement, and evaluate the care of patients after graduation from a school of nursing.

c. Discharge outcomes. Discharge outcomes often appear at the end of critical pathways used with hospitalized patients. They usually are achievable by most patients in several days to a week, depending on the medical diagnosis. Intermediate or daily outcomes that patients achieve during recovery advance them to these discharge outcomes. Discharge outcomes for a patient having a total knee replacement might be expected to be achieved in 5 days. These outcomes identify the behavior the patient is expected to achieve to be safely discharged from the institution. The patient then may go home and continue recovering independently or may need continuing care from a home health agency. The patient may go to an extended care facility or nursing home for further recovery and treatment. Each agency providing care generally has discharge outcomes that patients meet to advance safely to a less intense level of care until total independence is achieved. If patients are unable to achieve discharge outcomes, they may remain in the facility longer or permanently. Even within a hospital, areas such as the postanesthesia recovery room (PAR) and the intensive care unit (ICU) often have discharge outcomes for their acute-care areas. When patients are able to achieve these outcomes, they are advanced to a less acute-care setting, often going to a room on a medical-surgical floor. For example, discharge outcomes from the PAR after surgery with general anesthesia might include the following:

Spontaneous respirations in the normal adult range.
Arousable with stimulation.
Return of the swallow-gag reflex.
Vital signs in the normal range for this patient.
Pain rated at a level of 5 or less.

When patients achieve these outcomes, they are transferred out of the PAR and admitted to a room on one of the postsurgical stations of the hospital. To be discharged from the hospital, a patient will be expected to meet discharge outcomes that reflect the normal recovery progress and a level of functioning that can safely be cared for in a less acute setting. For example, to be discharged to the home from the hospital after a total knee replacement, a patient might be expected to meet the following outcomes:

States that pain management is acceptable on oral analgesics.
VS within normal range for individual.
Range of motion in knee up to 80 degrees of flexion or more.
Walks 50 feet demonstrating correct technique for crutch cane or walking.
Climbs up and down three stairs using correct crutch walking or cane.
No signs and symptoms of wound infection or delayed healing at incision site.

Inability to achieve any of these outcomes may result in a delayed discharge or transfer to an extended care facility rather than to the home.

Some outcomes are designed to maintain a continuous level of functioning during the time the patient is receiving nursing care. These outcomes usually are related to at-risk rather than actual nursing diagnoses. They do not have a specified time for achievement but imply systematic assessment and evaluation for as long as the risk for the problem developing exists. These outcomes span several days to weeks or more. For example:

1. Patient to report that pain is controlled at an acceptable level during hospitalization.
2. Patient to report that pain remains below 4 on a 1–10 scale during the postoperative period.
3. Skin integrity maintained during hospitalization.
4. Normal breath sounds maintained during postoperative period.
5. Maintenance of body weight between 135 and 140 lbs (forever).

These outcomes would be evaluated periodically as part of the plan of care rather than having a set time or date for evaluation as with the other outcomes discussed. For example (see outcomes above):

1. Assess pain every 3 to 4 hours.
2. Assess pain on 1–10 scale every 3 to 4 hours.
3. Assess skin integrity every 2 hours.
4. Assess breath sounds every 4 hours.
5. Assess body weight every morning or once a week.

These assessments would then be documented in the patient's chart until the risk for the problem was eliminated.

d. Health promotion/wellness outcomes.   Once outcomes to restore functioning or the previous level of health have been reached, the nurse is alert to the

opportunity to help patients and their families find ways to stay healthy. It is cheaper in terms of money and energy to live in a way that encourages health than it is to treat illnesses and injuries. Just having been ill or injured and now having recovered is an excellent motivator for people to try to live healthier, safer lives. Helping people make changes in how they live, their habits, and the risks they take is a primary responsibility for nurses in the area of health promotion and lifelong wellness. That first heart attack is a great motivator to quit smoking, lose weight, and get more exercise. Patients and families will need help in knowing how to live in a more health-promoting manner. Some lifelong wellness outcomes might include the following:

Physical well-being: freedom from injury, illness, and disease.
Active involvement in life, physically, mentally, and emotionally from birth to death.
Psychosocial well-being: strong self-esteem and social support system.
Balance of life roles: personal, family, career.
Reports feeling healthy, useful, and happy in all growth and development stages.
Stress rating low with life satisfaction rating high.

Guidelines for Writing Outcome Statements

In learning to write outcomes based on nursing diagnoses, consider the following criteria:

1. **For an actual nursing diagnosis, the outcome is a patient behavior that demonstrates reduction or alleviation of the problem.** Start with the nursing diagnosis. What is the problem? If the nursing diagnosis is "Acute pain related to broken right arm as evidenced by patient's report, crying, and elevated pulse," the outcome will demonstrate alleviation or lessening of the pain (not healing of the arm). If the nursing diagnosis is "Constipation related to dehydration and use of analgesics with codeine," the outcome deals with bowel elimination patterns showing restoration of normal function (not improved hydration or limiting the amount of codeine). The examples in Table 4-1 demonstrate the relationship between the nursing diagnosis and the outcome. A general nursing diagnostic category from the NANDA list is presented first, with individualized diagnostic statements underneath. Two formats are used for the diagnostic statement of actual nursing diagnoses: the three-part statement and the two-part statement with supporting data underneath. A long-term outcome and one or more intermediate goals are identified for each diagnosis.

2. **For at-risk nursing diagnoses, the outcome is a patient behavior that demonstrates maintenance of the current status of health or functioning.** If the potential nursing diagnosis is "Impaired skin integrity: high risk, related to casting of left leg," the outcome will demonstrate maintenance

OUTCOME STATEMENTS

Patient Behavior	+ Criteria	+ Time	+ Condition (if relevant)
Weight gain	of ½ ounce	every day until discharge	on 24 calorie/oz formula.
Weight pain	of ¼ ounce	every day until discharge	on breast-feeding with no supplement.
Self-injection	of correct insulin dose, using sterile technique	by November 4	using an autoinjector.
Maintenance of joint mobility	at current level	while on bed rest.	
Regain	15 lbs	in 2 months	on 2300-cal. diet and twice-daily insulin injections.
Oral intake	of 500 ml	by 3 P.M.	without abdominal distension, nausea, or vomiting.
Report pain reduced	at a level of 4 or less	during the first 24 hrs postop	with morphine PCA.
Report pain reduced	at a level of 4 or less	during 24 hrs–48 hrs postop	with the use of oral analgesics q3–4 hours prn.
Will void	at least 300 cc	before bladder becomes distended.	
Will void	at least 200 cc	within 6 hours	after removal of Foley catheter.

TABLE 4-1   RELATIONSHIP OF THE DIAGNOSIS TO THE OUTCOMES

Nursing Diagnoses	Outcomes
*Constipation related to dehydration and bed rest as evidenced by hard-to-pass stool and no BM for 5 days	Reestablish normal bowel pattern by discharge ∘ bowel movement by 3 P.M. today after Fleet enema
• Constipation related to dehydration and bed rest Supporting data: no BM for 5 days, reports stool hard to pass	∘ bowel movement tomorrow without use of enema
*Pain related to tissue trauma secondary to surgery as evidenced by rating pain as 8, elevated pulse, and BP 136/72	Report of negligible pain by discharge ∘ pain reported at a level of 3 or less within the next hour
• Pain related to tissue trauma secondary to surgery Supporting data: pulse 92, BP 136/72, pain rated as 8	∘ pain reduced to a level of 3 or less during the next 24 hours with IM analgesics ∘ pain reduced to a level of 3 or less after 48 hours postop with oral analgesic
*Ineffective airway clearance: related to weakness and lowered level of consciousness as evidenced by inability to remove secretions from back of throat	Independent maintenance of clear airway by 3/8 ∘ airway free of tracheal mucus within next ½ hour ∘ productive cough by 12 hours ∘ clear breath sounds in 24 hours
• Ineffective airway clearance related to weakness and lowered LOC Supporting data: O_2 sat. 88% on 2L O_2; weakness, gurgling of mucus in throat; difficult to arouse; 86 years old; 1 hour postop, no coughing.	

* = PES format (problem + etiology + signs/symptoms)

• = problem + etiology format

∘ = intermediate outcomes

of intact skin (not healing of the leg). If the nursing diagnosis is "High risk for impaired thermoregulation related to newborn status," the outcome demonstrates maintenance of the newborn's temperature in the normal range.

3. **The outcome is realistic for the patient's capabilities in the time span you designate in your outcome.** An outcome for a preterm baby weighing 4 pounds that stated, "Baby will weigh 8 pounds at the end of 1 week," would be unrealistic for this newborn. But if the outcome stated, "Baby will weigh 4 1/2 pounds in 7 days," the capabilities of the patient would have been considered and would make the outcome more realistic and more likely to be achieved. Experience, professional literature, references, the use of a critical pathway, and advice from other, more experienced nurses will help the student learn what is realistic for patients with particular problems.

4. **The outcome is realistic for the nurse's level of skill, experience, and time/workload.** If the nursing diagnosis is dealing with a problem beyond the nurse's role, the best course of action is to refer the problem to the appropriate professional. A patient with a nursing diagnosis of "Altered nutrition: less than body requirements related to refusal to eat hospital food as evidenced by 5-lb weight loss" is referred to a dietitian. A patient with a nursing diagnosis of "Impaired verbal communication related to recent stroke as evidenced by inability to say any word except *no*" is referred to a speech therapist when the patient's condition is sufficiently stable.

5. **The outcome is congruent with and supportive of other therapies.** This means that outcomes for the patient do not contradict or interfere with the work of other professionals caring for the patient. If the nursing diagnosis is "Urinary retention related to decreased urge, and perineal swelling as evidenced by residual urine volumes over 500 cc × 2," an intermediate outcome to have the patient void 300 cc this shift would be in conflict with a medical order to leave the catheter in place for 12 hours if the second residual urine was more than 200 cc.

6. **Whenever possible, the outcome is important and valued by the patient and family, the nurses, and the physician.** If outcomes are important to patients, they will be more motivated to reach them. If nurses value the outcomes, they will be more likely to carry out the suggested plan of care. The physician's understanding and support of nursing outcomes will help assure congruence with medical treatment. The outcomes also serve as a communication tool that keeps health team members informed about the patient's progress.

7. **The outcome is an observable or measurable patient behavior.** This means the nurse can see, hear, feel, or measure the patient's response. Try to avoid words such as *good, normal, adequate,* and *improved.* These words mean different things to different people and tend to make the outcome unclear. There may be disagreement about whether the outcome was achieved if words requiring a judgment are used in the outcome statement.

Remember, the nurse cannot see a patient "understanding," "feeling," or "knowing about."

Observable Verbs

reports	eats	sleeps
walks	drinks	breathes
rates	voids	demonstrates

Observable Outcomes	*Vague Outcomes*
The patient will walk the length of the hall unassisted by 2/5.	Increased ambulation or Adequate leg strength
Patient will gain ¼ lb each week until discharged.	Increased intake or Good nutrition or Promote weight gain

8. Write outcomes in terms of patient behavior, not nursing actions.

Patient Outcomes	*Nursing Actions*
The patient will void by 6 P.M.	I will offer the patient the urinal every 2 hours.
The patient will safely bathe her baby before she is discharged.	I will show the patient a baby bath before she is discharged.
The patient's temperature will be up to 98° F within 1 hour.	I will put warm blankets and a heating pad on the patient and recheck his temperature in 1 hour.

9. Keep the outcome short.
10. Make the outcome specific.
11. Derive each outcome from only one nursing diagnosis.
12. Designate a specific time for the achievement of each outcome.

CLASSIFICATION OF NURSING OUTCOMES

A large research team from the University of Iowa has developed a classification of patient outcomes that are achievable primarily through nursing interventions. The team's work is presented in the text *Nursing Outcomes Classification (NOC)* (Mosby, 1997), which contains 190 outcomes with specific indicators (patient behaviors) on a 1–5 rating scale that nurses can use to evaluate the

effectiveness of nursing interventions. Each outcome has a name, a definition, and a set of patient behaviors to use as evidence of outcome achievement or progress (or lack of progress) toward achievement. This text complements the other text developed by researchers from the Iowa Intervention Project, *Nursing Interventions Classification (NIC)* (Mosby, 1996). This text is a classification of nursing interventions to reduce or eliminate the problems identified by nursing diagnoses. Both the NOC outcomes and the NIC interventions are linked to NANDA nursing diagnoses for easier use in these phases of the nursing process. An example of this work is included in this chapter and in Chapter 5, where interventions are discussed. Pain was chosen as the nursing diagnosis to follow through NOC outcomes (Table 4-2 and 4-3) and NIC interventions (Tables 5-2

TABLE 4-2   DIAGNOSES, OUTCOMES, AND INTERVENTIONS

NANDA nursing diagnosis: Pain
Definition: a state in which an individual experiences and reports the presence of severe discomfort or an uncomfortable sensation

NOC-Suggested Nursing Outcomes for Pain Resolution

Outcome Classification	Definition
Comfort Level	Feelings of physical and psychological ease
Pain Control Behavior	Personal actions to control pain
Pain: Disruptive Effects	Observed or reported disruptive effects of pain on emotions and behavior
Pain Level	Amount of reported or demonstrated pain

NIC-Suggested Initial Nursing Interventions for Pain Resolution

Intervention	Definition
Analgesic Administration	Use of pharmacological agents to reduce or eliminate pain
Conscious Sedation	Administration of sedatives, monitoring of the patient's response, and provision of necessary physiological support during diagnostic or therapeutic procedures
Pain Management	Alleviation of pain or reduction in pain to a level of comfort that is acceptable to the patient
Patient-Controlled Analgesia (PCA) Assistance	Facilitating patient control of analgesic administration and regulation

Source: Adapted from Johnson, M., Maas, M., (1997) *Nursing Outcomes Classification (NOC)*, St. Louis: Mosby; McCloskey, J., Bulechek, G., (1996) *Nursing Interventions Classification (NIC)*, 2nd ed., St. Louis: Mosby. Used by permission.

TABLE 4-3 NURSING OUTCOMES CLASSIFICATION (NOC): PAIN CONTROL
BEHAVIOR DEFINITION: PERSONAL ACTIONS TO CONTROL PAIN

Indicators: Rated on a 1 (never demonstrated) to 5 (consistently demonstrated)
scale

	1	2	3	4	5
Recognizes causal factors					
Recognizes pain onset					
Uses preventive technique					
Uses nonanalgesic relief measures					
Uses analgesics appropriately					
Uses warning signs to seek care					
Reports symptoms to health care professional					
Uses available resources					
Recognizes symptoms of pain					
Uses pain diary					
Reports pain control					
Other _____ (specify)					

From Johnson, M., Maas M., (1997) *Nursing Outcomes Classification (NOC)*, St. Louis: Mosby.
Used by permission.

and 5-3) because of the universality of this problem in all areas of nursing practice and patient care.

CRITICAL THINKING FOR OUTCOME IDENTIFICATION

In setting priorities and selecting outcomes, a nurse uses critical thinking by combining knowledge, experience, and reasoning to create realistic, individualized outcomes for each unique patient. The relationship between the diagnosis and the outcomes must be clearly understood so that the outcomes achieve the purpose of showing a reduction or improvement in or prevention of the problem identified in the diagnosis. These outcomes then serve as standards against which to evaluate the patient's response to nursing care. This is another skill in critical thinking and problem solving. Multiple factors are considered, including age, family situation, living arrangements, culture, and strengths and resources, as the nurse creatively matches an outcome to a patient's nursing diagnosis. The textbook outcome for a poorly controlled diabetic patient might be accurate assessment of blood glucose four times a day. In reality, the outcome for this homeless patient with few supplies might be to check glucose once a week since

at present she checks her glucose only once a month. A critically thinking nurse views patients within their actual context and is reality-based. This type of nurse shows mature thinking by accepting that things are not always perfect. Any improvement is a worthy outcome and is more likely to be acceptable to this patient.

A critically thinking nurse is aware of personal biases in setting priorities. Is the patient seeing this nursing diagnosis as a priority too? Being open-minded, knowing there are many ways to look at a problem, and having the perseverance to keep trying are characteristics of critical thinkers that are important in the outcome identification phase of the nursing process.

Textbook knowledge and clinical experience are combined with knowledge of this patient, family, and culture in the reasoning processes of the nurse as outcomes are selected. What are most patients in this situation able to do and when? What behavior would be best for this patient to show progress toward problem resolution? What is a realistic criterion of performance and time frame for this patient on the basis of my assessment? This all requires purposeful, disciplined, reflective reasoning, that is, critical thinking.

Prompts for Critical Thinking During Outcome Identification

- Could you have missed or underestimated any priorities because of personal biases?
- What does the patient think is a priority outcome? The family? Other care providers?
- Do the outcomes clearly show improvement, resolution, or prevention of the problem?
- Are the outcomes culturally sensitive? Age-appropriate?
- What level of health does this patient want by tomorrow, by discharge, in a month?
- What are the expected outcomes for most patients with this medical problem? Are yours congruent?
- What outcomes must be at least minimally achieved for patient safety?
- Are the criteria selected for the outcome clear, observable or measurable, and realistic?

CULTURALLY COMPETENT NURSING CARE DURING OUTCOME IDENTIFICATION

The 1998 American Nurses Association *Standards of Clinical Nursing Practice* states, "Outcomes are culturally appropriate." This is part of nursing's goal of

individualized care. Our culture is part of who we are as individuals. Our cultural view of what health and illness are affect which health goals we think are appropriate. Outcomes developed without consideration for the patient's cultural beliefs, values, and practices may seem inappropriate to the patient; a patient is likely to be noncompliant with a plan developed to achieve those outcomes. What outcome is important for this patient in this culture?

The dominant U.S. health care culture believes that breast-feeding a newborn frequently during the first 24 to 48 hours of life is important for success. Some cultures believe that it is not appropriate to start breast-feeding until the milk comes in a few days after delivery. These grandmas tell the nurse, "No, no, no milk yet," when attempts are made to get their daughters to nurse their newborns. What is a nurse to do when the lactation policy or breast-feeding clinical pathway is to have new mothers feed every 2 to 4 hours around the clock? Lighten up. The nurse's way is only one way. The outcome of successful breast-feeding is important to everyone, but cultural norms around birth and feeding are very important. The role of the grandmother in guiding the new mother also may have cultural norms. The nurse does not discredit the grandmother by imposing Western medicine's standard breast-feeding pathway. That would show disrespect. Strike a balance: Once or twice versus every 3 hours probably is much more acceptable "just to give the new mom practice." The nurse thus acknowledges the grandmother's knowledge and skill in helping her daughter.

Prompts for Culturally Competent Nursing Care During Outcome Identification

- What level of problem resolution would make the patient feel ready to go home?
- Is the outcome congruent with the patient's cultural views of appropriate behavior in the sick role?
- Is the outcome viewed as "good" or "harmful" for eventual recovery on the basis of cultural expectations for the course of illness and its treatment?
- How can outcomes developed for Anglo-Americans be adapted to fit other cultures?

PATIENT OUTCOMES: THE MANAGED CARE ENVIRONMENT

Within the managed care environment, there are two broad classifications of patient outcomes that are of concern to nurses and patients: clinical outcomes and fiscal outcomes. Clearly, no one would deny that the clinical outcomes of patients are the most important and primary focus of nurses and other health care

providers. However, few nurses understand what fiscal outcomes mean to patients, health care institutions, and the survival of the profession of nursing.

Clinical outcomes have been described in this chapter as the desired result of nursing care. Nurses identify outcomes for physiological, psychosocial, and spiritual needs. Many outcomes are identified as a result of a surgical procedure or disease condition. These outcomes might include a pain level or safety in crutch walking for a patient having orthopedic surgery. These clinical outcomes will be the same for all patients who undergo the same procedure. Other outcomes are highly individualized. For example, the patient with the orthopedic procedure may be the single parent of a toddler. This patient may have nursing diagnoses related to her parenting role and ability to care for an active child. In this case the nurse may begin care by using the standardized patient outcomes for orthopedic surgery but then individualize those outcomes to meet the unique needs of this patient. Both the standardized outcomes and the unique patient outcomes are essential for high-quality patient care.

Sometimes you may hear the term *nursing-sensitive patient outcomes*. This term refers to patient outcomes that are directly affected by nursing care. It is well established in nursing research that maintaining skin integrity in elderly, bedridden patients is affected by positioning, nutrition, massage, and personal hygiene. Thus, the outcome of maintaining intact skin is a nursing-sensitive patient outcome. Nurse researchers are beginning to publish studies that demonstrate that the achievement of these patient outcomes is dependent on adequate staffing levels of registered nurses. As a profession, nurses need to understand when patients' clinical outcomes may be jeopardized.

Fiscal outcomes of care are also important to both the patient and the institution. Fiscal outcomes are outcomes that have to do with financial matters. The first obligation of the nurse is to the patient. If the patient is required to remain in the hospital an extra day or two because an acceptable discharge plan was not established, the patient or the patient's insurance company may receive an unnecessary bill. This may result from poor communication between physicians, nurses, case managers, and social workers. An example would be a situation in which a decision is made to discharge the patient to a nursing home. This process may take several days to have the family select a facility, make financial arrangements, and complete the necessary paperwork. The insurance company may decline to pay for those hospital days because it was not necessary for the patient to be cared for in the hospital; it was established that the patient was ready to move to a lower level of care. If this results in the patient receiving a bill, a negative fiscal outcome has occurred that could have been prevented.

There are also fiscal outcomes for the institution. Most hospitals, for example, know that there is a dollar amount that it costs to provide certain services. Hospital managers may have established that it costs about $4000 to care for a woman with a 2-day hospitalization (length of stay, or LOS) for a vaginal hysterectomy. When these managers review monthly data, if they see that the cost has increased to $5000 and most patients have been staying 3 to 4 days, they begin to investigate. Is there something different about the care of these women?

Was there an increase in the cost of surgical supplies? Was there a high rate of infection that required a longer length of stay? Often these fiscal outcomes are a signal of clinical issues. However, if this trend of increasing costs continues indefinitely, it will be difficult for the hospital to meet its expenses (one expense is paying nurses' salaries) and stay in business.

Nurses' first accountability is always to achieve the clinical outcomes of patient care. However, coupling clinical and fiscal outcomes is a skill required of nurses in the managed care environment. It is another way we meet our responsibilities to our patients.

SUMMARY

During the outcome identification phase of the nursing process, the nurse and the patient set priorities among the identified problems and establish outcomes showing reduction, prevention, or elimination of the problem. An outcome is the desired behavioral change in the patient after nursing care. For actual nursing diagnoses, the outcomes identify patient behavior demonstrating a lessening or elimination of the problem. For high-risk nursing diagnoses, the outcomes demonstrate that patients are maintaining the current level of functioning or preventing the problem from developing. Outcomes give direction to nursing actions as do nursing diagnoses. Longer-term outcomes, also called final outcomes or discharge outcomes, demonstrate the maximum level of functioning for the patient or restoration of normal functioning and may take days to months to achieve. Intermediate outcomes describe patient behavior in smaller steps. They may be more appropriate in a hospital where the patient stays only a few days or in a more critical care setting when the patient is unstable and the problem must be reduced or eliminated rapidly. Intermediate outcomes may be set in a time frame of hours to days. They are progressive and are used to show continued advancement, in terms of improved level of patient functioning, in the direction of long-term or discharge outcome. An outcome statement contains the patient behavior, the criteria for acceptable performance of that behavior, the time frame in which the outcome should be achieved, and the conditions, if any, under which the behavior will be demonstrated. Outcomes are realistic, observable, congruent with other health professionals' plans of care, and directly related to the nursing diagnosis.

PRACTICE EXERCISE

Pick out the correctly written outcomes. Identify what is wrong with the incorrectly written ones. The answers follow the exercise.

1. The patient's hydration will improve.
2. The nurse will reduce the patient's anxiety.

3. The patient will know about infant feeding.
4. Improve muscle strength.
5. 3/5: The patient will lose 6 lbs in 2 weeks.
6. The patient will talk about her labor within 24 hours after delivery.
7. The decubitus ulcer (bed sore) will be healed by 2/5.
8. Verbalization of decreased pain within the next hour.
9. The patient will express confidence in her ability to breast-feed her baby before discharge.
10. Turn and deep breathe the patient every 2 hours.
11. Ankle edema will decrease.
12. The patient will feel better by bedtime.
13. The patient will ambulate.
14. Teach the patient AROM (active range of motion) exercises.
15. The patient's depression will improve.
16. The patient will learn about good nutrition.
17. The patient will understand the purpose of his or her medications before discharge.
18. The patient's temperature will stay below 101° F during the next 24 hours.
19. The nursing student will understand the nursing process after reading this book.
20. The student will write a nursing diagnosis and final (long-term) outcome with two intermediate outcomes after finishing this chapter.

ANSWERS TO EXERCISE ON OUTCOME STATEMENTS

1. Not specific or observable. A better outcome would be:
The patient's intake will be 2500 cc every 24 hours.
or
The patient will drink at least 75 cc each hour.
2. Not observable. This is a nurse behavior instead of a patient behavior. No time limit is set. A better outcome would be:
Verbalization of reduced anxiety about tomorrow's surgery by 10 P.M. tonight.
or
The patient will discuss feelings related to biopsy by 3 P.M. today.
3. Not observable, no time limit. A better outcome would be:
States how to prepare formula by discharge.
or
Newborn regained birth weight on breast milk by 2-week checkup.
4. No subject, not specific, no criteria. A better outcome would be:
The patient will lift his own weight using the bed trapeze by 2/5.
or

4/5: The patient will lift equal amounts of weight in 3 months with his right arm and his left arm.

5. OK.
6. OK.
7. OK.
8. Subject (the patient) is assumed. Is any decrease in pain acceptable for the achievement of this intermediate outcome? If pain goes from "unbearable" to "very severe," would you be satisfied? Would the patient? Better outcome: Pain rated as 3 or less at the end of 1 hour.
9. OK.
10. This is a nursing action, not an observable patient behavior.
11. Not specific, no time limit. A better outcome would be:
Absence of edema of the ankle by tomorrow at 10 P.M.
or
Ankle will measure 10 inches in circumference or less by tomorrow at 8 A.M.
12. Not observable. A better outcome would be:
The patient will state that anxiety about being hospitalized has decreased by h.s.
13. No criteria. A better outcome would be:
The patient will walk the length of the hall by the date of discharge without the use of a walker.
or
8/2: The patient will walk from his or her bed to a chair in the room by tomorrow.
14. Nursing action instead of patient behavior, no time limit. A better outcome would be:
The patient will demonstrate AROM by 3 P.M. today.
or
The patient will have equal motion in the right shoulder and left shoulder joint by the time of discharge.
15. Too vague, not observable. A better outcome would be:
The patient will sit in patient lounge for 15 minutes during this shift.
or
8/3: The patient will get dressed and comb her or his hair tomorrow A.M.
16. Not observable. A better outcome would be:
(The patient) Select a food from each of the four basic food groups for tonight's supper.
or
(The patient) Plan a week's menu for a low-salt diet with the help of the dietitian before discharge.
17. Not observable. A better outcome would be:
The patient will state the purpose of each of his or her medications before discharge.
or

By 4/7, the patient will state route, dose, and time for each take-home medication.
18. OK.
19. Not observable. A better outcome would be:
The nursing student will list the steps in the nursing process after reading this book.
or
The nursing student will write one nursing care plan after reading this book.
20. OK.

CASE STUDY: OUTCOME IDENTIFICATION

The case study of Mrs. Wiley is continued from Chapter 3 to identify clinical outcomes of the care process.

PATIENT OUTCOMES #1
PREOPERATIVE ORTHOPEDIC SURGERY CLINIC

Mrs. Wiley: Clinical outcomes are identified by the nurse in the orthopedic clinic.

Nursing Diagnosis	Clinical Outcomes
Knowledge deficit: strengthening exercises, crutch walking, pain management after surgery, use of incentive spirometer, preoperative preparation for surgery	Verbalize/demonstrate: strengthening exercises, anticipated length of stay, what to expect during hospitalization, understanding of pain management (PCA) and pain rating scale, use of incentive spirometer, crutch walking before surgery.
Husband: risk for injury related to absence of care provider	Husband will remain free of injury during absence and recovery of primary caregiver (Mrs. Wiley).
Chronic pain related to degeneration of knee joint	Patient will state that pain is controlled at 4 or less on activity or less than 2 at rest until the time of surgery.

PATIENT OUTCOMES #2
FIRST DAY SURGERY CENTER: 6 A.M.

Patients are admitted to the first day surgery center the morning of surgery for their scheduled procedures and are transferred to the inpatient unit after surgery.

Mrs. Wiley: Clinical outcomes are identified by the nurse at the time of admission, 6 A.M. on the day of surgery.

Nursing Diagnosis	Clinical Outcomes
Fear of reduced mobility related to outcome of surgery	Patient will report reduced fear level before leaving preop area.
Risk for injury (Mrs. Wiley) related to lack of experience in crutch walking	Patient will be injury-free during hospitalization and home recovery.
Anxiety (patient and family members) related to surgical experience	Patient and family will demonstrate reduced anxiety within 6 hours as evidenced by: patient or family will state relief at outcomes of surgery.

PATIENT OUTCOMES #3
POSTOPERATIVE ORTHOPEDIC PATIENT CARE UNIT

Mrs. Wiley: Clinical outcomes are identified by the nurse during the first hours after surgery.

Nursing Diagnosis	Clinical Outcomes
Acute pain related to joint replacement therapy, physical therapy, and movement	Pain will remain at 3 or less throughout hospitalization.
Risk for caregiver role strain (upon discharge) related to dependency of frail spouse and surgery of caregiver	Caregiver and husband will identify needs at home and plan assistance during care planning conference before discharge.

(continued)

| Impaired physical mobility, level 2*, related to knee replacement surgery | Patient will manage independent ambulation and stair climbing with crutches by discharge. |
| Risk for injury (Mrs. Wiley) related to lack of experience with crutch walking | Patient will remain free of falls during hospitalization and home recovery. |

PATIENT OUTCOMES #4
HOME HEALTH CARE AGENCY

Mrs. Wiley: Clinical outcomes are identified by the nurse at the time of the first home visit.

Nursing Diagnosis	Clinical Outcomes
Knowledge/skill deficit: signs/symptoms to report to MD; aseptic technique; self-administered medication, purpose, schedule; wound care; pain management techniques	Reports elevated temperature/chills to MD within 2 hours. Attains healing of wound without complications within 14 days Demonstrates aseptic technique during wound care by second visit. Maintains pain at 2 or less during week 1 at home.
Acute pain related to joint replacement surgery, physical therapy, and movement	Pain at 1–2 rating with movement.
Risk for injury (Mrs. Wiley) related to lack of experience with crutch walking	Remains free of falls at home.

* Requires help from another person for assistance, supervision, or teaching.

CHAPTER 5

Planning

STANDARD IV. PLANNING

The Nurse Develops a Plan of Care That Prescribes Interventions to Attain Expected Outcomes.

Reprinted with permission from American Nurses Association, *Standards of Clinical Nursing Practice*, 2nd edition, © 1998 American Nurses Publishing, American Nurses Foundation/ American Nurses Association, Washington, D.C.

Nursing interventions are activities that the nurse plans and implements to help a patient achieve identified outcomes. By achieving these outcomes, the patient will reduce or eliminate the diagnosed problems. Nursing interventions may be referred to in several ways: nursing actions, nursing strategies, nursing treatment plans, and nursing orders. This text will use all these terms to mean the same things. Some texts uses the term *nursing interventions* to mean a general activity such as "force fluids," and a *nursing action or order* then refers to a specific, individualized activity, such as "100 cc fluids q2h × next 24°." The nurse, using a problem-solving approach, selects activities to do with and for the patient that are most likely to result in achievement of the outcome. There are many nursing interventions from which to choose to help reduce a given problem. The nurse tries to select the best ones, based on the desired outcome, patient abilities and preferences, available resources, nursing knowledge and experience, and the protocols of the health care facility.

The planned nursing interventions are communicated to other nurses on the patient's care plan to promote a consistent approach toward the achievement of an outcome. Often the nurse who has the most information about the patient and expertise in the particular problem areas diagnosed is the one who selects the most appropriate nursing interventions. The written care plan communicates this plan for outcome achievement to others who will provide 24-hour nursing care. The nursing interventions written on the patient's care plan are instructions for others to follow, since they may not have the knowledge of or experience with the patient that the original nurse gained during the assessment phase.

Nursing interventions are similar to physician's orders since they specify a plan of care aimed at achieving an outcome. For others to follow a plan of care, it must be specific or it may be interpreted inappropriately. Interventions should identify

—what is to be done
—when the activity is to be done and how often
—the duration for each intervention, when appropriate
—any preceding or follow-up activities
—the date interventions were selected
—the sequence in which nursing activities are to be performed when one activity is dependent on or facilitated by a previous action
—signature or initials of the nurse writing the plan of care

When these things are identified by the professional nurse on a patient's plan of nursing care, other nurses are held responsible and accountable to the patient, nurse colleagues, and the health care facility for the prescribed care. Other nurses know to whom to direct questions regarding the patient. They know to whom to direct feedback regarding patient responses following the prescribed care. Physicians may seek out the nurse who wrote the plan of care for a patient as the person most knowledgeable about that patient's response to ordered treatments. All of this may seem somewhat threatening to a student in nursing who may feel unsure of his or her ability to identify accurate diagnoses, select appropriate outcomes, and choose nursing interventions most likely to achieve those outcomes. It is a learning process, but without both positive and negative feedback from other nurses who carry out the plan, students will not improve their skills in planning patient care.

NURSING INTERVENTIONS:

Those specific activities the nurse plans and implements to help the patient achieve an outcome.

TYPES OF NURSING INTERVENTIONS

There are several broad categories of nursing interventions. Combining actions from several different groups is often the most effective plan. These groupings of nursing interventions include the following.

Environmental Management

This aspect of nursing care involves establishing and maintaining a safe therapeutic environment. A noisy, cluttered, or stark environment is not the best

atmosphere to promote rest and recovery. Attention to room order, opening and closing curtains for light, wall calendars showing the correct date, opening and reading mail, and keeping the bed clean and straightened and the nightstand accessible with needed personal articles are all activities that fall into this category. These activities may not require the expertise of a professional nurse, but it may be the nurse's responsibility to help with or delegate these activities. The patient and family may be uneasy in a health care setting where no one attends to environmental management.

"Very few people . . . have any idea of the exquisite cleanliness required in the sick room. . . . The well have a curious habit of forgetting that what is to them but a trifling inconvenience, to be patiently "put up" with, is to the sick a source of suffering, delayed recovery, if not actually hastening death. The well are scarcely ever more than eight hours, at most, in the same room. Some change they can make, if only for a few minutes. . . . But the sick man who never leaves his bed, who cannot change by any movement of his own his air, or his light, or his warmth; who cannot obtain quiet, or get out of the smoke, or the dust; he is really poisoned or depressed by what is to you the merest trifle."   p. 92

Florence Nightingale, *Notes on Nursing: What It Is and What It Is Not*. From an unabridged republication of the first American edition as published in 1860. (1969) New York: Dover Publications.

Physician-Initiated and -Ordered Interventions

Based on the physician's diagnosis of the patient's health problems, orders to assess, schedule tests, and provide treatments will be written by the physician in the patient's chart. The nurse is expected to implement these orders. Implementation of these orders is still considered part of nursing interventions because the nurse individualizes the way the order is carried out based on the patient's status at the time. The nurse often explains what is to be done and why. The nurse may give the patient and family some choices within the scope of implementing the order. The timing of the implementation often is adjusted or designated by the professional nurse to fit in with constraints on personnel within the health care setting while still providing safety for the patient and performance of the ordered activity. An example is intravenous (IV) therapy. The physician orders the type and amount of fluid to infuse and the rate. The nurse often does the venipuncture, sets up the IV system, and keeps it running. The nurse assesses the patient response frequently and may discontinue the infusion if problems develop. The nurse may refer the problem to a specially trained IV nurse to restart treatment. Based on other assessments of the patient, the nurse may discuss with the physician whether IV therapy is required since the patient is now

drinking well with good bowel sounds. Clinical pathways for various medical diagnoses have predetermined physician orders, outcomes, and nursing interventions set out on a time schedule. These orders often need to be individualized to the patient since they are developed for a "generic patient" rather than from an assessment of this patient.

Nurse-Initiated and Physician-Ordered Interventions

Based on the nurse's assessment of the patient and identification of problems, the nurse may request help from the physician in treatment. The nurse is not licensed to order certain treatments but recognizes when they may be needed. The nurse is requesting an intervention order from the physician to help reduce or treat the problem the nurse has identified. An order to catheterize a patient who is unable to void may be written after the nurse notifies the physician of the problem, supporting data, and ineffective interventions implemented thus far. This type of intervention is most common in working with a collaborative problem.

Another example of this type of intervention occurs when the nurse collaborates with the physician regarding an already written order. The nurse may have identified a change in patient status and is questioning whether an order should be implemented as written or whether the physician would like to change the order based on current patient status and needs. For example, the physician may have written the order to begin clear liquids postoperatively and to discontinue the IV when the current bag has infused. The patient is experiencing a variation from the normal postop course and is unable to take any fluids, is nauseated and vomiting, and has an increased pulse. To discontinue the IV at this point would not be prudent without updating the physician on the patient's response postop. The nurse requests the physician's help, identifies the alteration in patient status, and requests clarification of the original order.

The physician frequently writes orders to be implemented only if the need arises (prn orders). The nurse then identifies whether the problem develops, adapts the interventions to the patient's status, implements the adapted order, and documents the patient's response. This is the case when the physician writes prn orders for different forms of analgesia in a dosage range. The nurse and the patient determine need for the medication, intensity of pain, type of pain, and effectiveness of last analgesia, and the nurse selects the medication and dose most likely to meet the patient's need for pain relief.

Nurse-Initiated and -Ordered Interventions

These interventions are solely in the range of professional nursing. The nurse assesses the patient, makes a nursing diagnosis, selects interventions, and implements those interventions or delegates implementation to other nursing personnel.

Within this category are several forms of independent nursing interventions:

1. Health teaching and health promotion.
2. Health counseling to help patients make informed choices.
3. Referrals to other nurses or health care professionals; transfer summaries to other stations, hospitals, or nursing homes; public health referrals; home health agency referrals.
4. Specific nursing treatments to prevent problems or lessen current difficulties, such as ambulating, turning and repositioning, suctioning the airway, feedings, cleaning and dressing a wound, range of motion exercises, optimum nutrition.
5. Providing support, comfort, and encouragement.
6. Assessment of patient status or response to treatments ordered by nurses, physicians, or other health professionals.
7. Discharge planning related to life-style changes, coping with health changes and medical treatments, and setting priorities. Examples might include

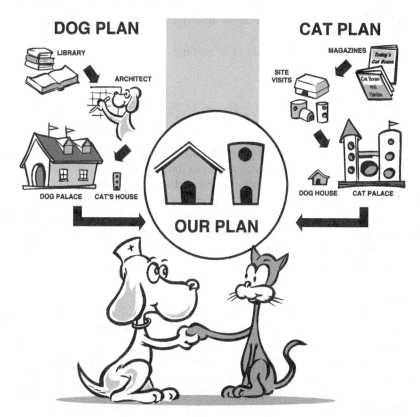

FIGURE 5-1.   The best plans are those that are mutually developed to meet the needs of all involved.

problem solving with a new diabetic patient and family on how to fit blood glucose monitoring, insulin injections, and food intake into a job requiring frequent travel and eating in restaurants.

8. Assistance with meeting basic needs/activities of daily living and ensuring safety.

Some examples of nursing interventions are the following:
INTERMEDIATE OUTCOME: Reestablish urinary elimination, with complete emptying of the bladder within 6 hours of removal of catheter.

Interventions:
- Offer assistance to the bathroom for voiding every 2 hours
- Encourage fluids, 1 glass of juice, every hour
- Record intake and output for 24 hours
- Offer analgesics every 3 to 4 hours
- Provide privacy for voiding attempts
- Run water in bathroom for voiding attempts
- Encourage application of pressure over bladder during voiding attempts
- Encourage voiding attempt in sitz bath, tub bath, or shower if unable to void in 5 hours
- Assess bladder for emptying after voiding

RATIONALE FOR NURSING INTERVENTIONS

Nursing actions are based on principles and knowledge integrated from previous nursing education and experience and from the behavioral and physical sciences. These principles identify the relationship between the nursing intervention and the achievement of outcomes. Nursing actions are known to affect people in predictable ways and are chosen to help a patient achieve those expected outcomes. For example, the effects of heat and cold applied to the skin are understood by the nurse. If the nurse wants to increase the blood flow to an area of the body as one way of promoting intermediate outcome achievement, a nursing intervention such as "warm packs to right arm 20 minutes 4 times a day" may be chosen.

The first courses in many nursing programs involve the student in a study of the fundamentals of nursing practice. These fundamentals courses provide the student with the rationale for the steps of various skills and procedures in addition to teaching the motor aspects of the skill or procedure. To safely adapt nursing care to new situations, new equipment, and changing technology, the nurse must understand the rationale behind the choice of nursing actions. Principles and theories related to sterile technique, for example, have remained constant as equipment and materials have changed from reusable supplies to disposable. The nurse who understands the rationale behind sterile technique for various

procedures is more able to adapt nursing care to a particular patient by using any variety of equipment and supplies available. Principles and theories from disciplines related to nursing, such as anatomy, physiology, microbiology, psychology, and sociology, blend with nursing knowledge and experience to form an integrated base of knowledge that guides the nurse in planning patient care. While the nursing process involves an understanding of the rationale underlying nursing actions, it is not necessary to include this written rationale in documenting the care plan. However, the nursing process is incomplete and potentially unsafe unless nurses base their choices of nursing actions on an appropriate rationale. Rationales for nursing actions are included in the various care plans in this text as a teaching tool. In clinical settings, writing rationales for nursing actions consumes much time and space and therefore is inappropriate.

The following example illustrates the principles and theories from various disciplines on which the selection of appropriate nursing actions is based.
NURSING DIAGNOSIS: Sleep pattern disturbance related to hospitalization, pain, and traction as evidenced by inability to fall asleep, reports of fatigue.
INTERMEDIATE OUTCOME: Improve nighttime sleep to at least 4 hours tonight.
LONG-TERM OUTCOME: Sleeping 6 hours/night by discharge without sleeping medication.

Nursing Interventions	Rationale
a. Obtain a sleep history	a. Provides baseline data from which to assess activities that promote or interfere with sleep.
b. Assess for factors in the current environment that interfere with sleep and minimize if possible	b. Noise, heat, cold, too hard or soft a bed, roommates, and lights can all interfere with sleep.
c. Offer pain medication at HS	c. Pain can interfere with sleep.
d. Offer back rub at HS	d. Back rubs help relax muscles and give the patient time to talk about any concerns; relaxation and decreased anxiety facilitate sleep.
e. Help to reposition in traction	e. Good body alignment decreases strain on muscles and promotes comfort to facilitate sleep.
f. Encourage good sleep hygiene	
◦ no caffeine after noon meal	◦ caffeine is a stimulant
◦ limit cigarette smoking	◦ nicotine can stimulate CNS
◦ offer light snack before bed	◦ foods high in protein and L-tryptophan (milk) promote sleep
◦ help to follow usual routine for hygiene, time to retire	◦ normal habits from home are associated with a good sleeping pattern

PROBLEM SOLVING AND
SELECTING INTERVENTIONS

How does a nurse choose the most appropriate interventions? Some nurses just seem to "know" what to do to help a patient achieve an outcome. Others do things because "we have always done it this way." Still others rely on a standard care plan or clinical pathway designed for all patients with a similar problem to tell them what to do. Where does a student begin? Nursing students do not base care on intuition. They have to learn how to be effective nurses. That means applying the skills of problem solving to a particular patient's health problems and the environment in which nursing care is to be given. The following suggestions may be helpful in selecting interventions.

1. Review the nursing diagnosis so that the problem and the etiology (cause) of the problem are clear. For *actual problems*, try to reduce or eliminate the problem and the cause of the problem. If the cause cannot be reduced or eliminated, select interventions to minimize or eliminate the problematic signs and symptoms. For problems at risk of occurring, select interventions that reduce or eliminate the risk factors. If this is not possible, select interventions to prevent the problem from developing, delay its development, or reduce the severity of the problem when it does develop. For example, insulin-dependent diabetics are at risk for tissue damage in the legs and feet. Teaching good foot care and maintenance of blood glucose levels as close to normal as possible may delay or prevent this complication or make it less severe and more easily treated.
2. Examine the intermediate and final outcomes so that you know where you are going and know the steps to get there.
3. Consider all possible nursing activities that might help the patient achieve the outcome:
    —changes in the environment
    —activities for the patient and family to perform independently
    —activities to perform with the patient
    —activities to perform for the patient
    —assistance from other health care professionals
    —involvement of the patient's friends and family
    —changes in the nurse (increased knowledge and skill)
4. Use standard care plans and critical clinical pathways as guidelines for developing and planning a patient's nursing care. These standards provide the nurse with general guidelines for patients with particular medical diagnoses, diagnostic studies, or nursing diagnoses. They identify areas for assessment, possible patient problems to anticipate, and suggested outcomes and nursing interventions. They provide the student and the nurse with another resource for planning nursing interventions. These standard care plans do not replace the individualized care plan developed by the nurse.

Based on the knowledge about an individual patient, the medical management of health problems, the health care setting, and patient and family preferences and concerns, the nurse will fill out the etiology and signs and symptoms of the diagnosis. Next the nurse selects and individualizes outcomes from a list of possible outcomes, deletes inappropriate interventions, adds new interventions, and individualizes general interventions. These plans save the nurse time in rewriting common nursing interventions but do not replace the process of planning individualized care (see Table 5-3 later in this chapter).

5. Use the patient and patient's family as a source of possible nursing interventions. They may have many good suggestions for activities the patient can perform, with or without nursing assistance, to achieve a certain outcome, based on the patient's past experience and personal preferences. The nurse then uses personal knowledge and experience to incorporate some of these suggestions into a plan of care. This collaboration helps involve patients and their families in planning and implementing the type of nursing care they receive. By using the patient and family to help plan nursing interventions, the nurse considers patient preferences, and this usually leads to more effective interventions.

6. Use resources such as nursing fundamentals texts, medical-surgical nursing texts, and current journal articles. Use the policy and procedure manual on the clinical setting for information on what is to be done and how to do it in a particular setting.

7. Consider the advantages and disadvantages of possible nursing interventions and select those that meet the following criteria:

- **Nursing actions must be safe for the patient.** For example, application of heat to the skin will stimulate circulation, but excessive heat will burn. Nursing actions using heat must ensure that the patient is not burned. Exercising a patient's muscles and joints can be very beneficial; however, if muscles and joints are forced beyond the point of resistance or pain, the nurse can cause injuries.

- **Nursing actions must be congruent with other therapies.** For example, nursing actions must be selected within the safety range ordered by the physician. If the medical order reads "Aspirin (ASA), 2 tablets, q4h, prn," nursing actions cannot plan the administration of aspirin every 2 hours. If the physical therapist is instructing the patient in the use of a walker, the nurse also should use a walker in ambulating the patient.

- **Nursing actions selected are most likely to develop the behavior described in the outcome.** There may be many different nursing actions that would accomplish the same outcome. The nurse attempts to give the patient practice in the specific behavior stated in the outcome. For example:
  - NURSING DIAGNOSIS: Pain related to movement secondary to bone cancer.
  - OUTCOME: Verbalization of pain as less than 3 on a 1–10 scale during hospitalization.

Nursing Actions/Interventions	
May Achieve Outcome	*More Likely to Achieve Outcome*
a. Offer prescribed pain medication q3–4h prn	a. Assess patient's pain, timing, duration, intensity, and related activities q3–4h b. Administer analgesic 1/2 hour before physical therapy c. Administer analgesic q3h while awake d. Assess patient's current methods of dealing with pain and support if possible e. Discuss and practice alternative pain relief measures by March 1 　(1) Relaxation 　(2) Alternative sensory stimulation 　　— music 　　— tactile (massage, effleurage, menthol rubs, vibrators) 　　— heat/cold 　　— movies, TV, reading 　(3) Breathing techniques f. Discuss self-medication for pain by March 3 g. Discuss effectiveness of pain relief measures with physician and patient h. Encourage use of pain relief measures when discomfort *begins* rather than after it is intense

- **Nursing actions are realistic:**
  — for the patient. Consider age, physical strength, disease, willingness to change behavior, resources.
  — for the number of hospital staff. Will enough people consistently be available to carry out the nursing actions?
  — for the experience and ability of available staff. If most of the staff are unfamiliar with the nursing actions you are suggesting or disagree with them, there is a high probability that they will not be carried out.
  — for available equipment. If your nursing actions include the use of any equipment, it should be readily available and the hospital staff should be familiar with its use.
- **Nursing actions consider meeting lower level survival needs before higher level needs.** For example, the following sequence of nursing actions

deals with the current need for pain avoidance before asking the patient to deal with high-risk problems.

NURSING DIAGNOSIS: Risk for ineffective breathing pattern related to general anesthesia, postop pain.

OUTCOME: Normal respiratory rate and lung sounds by second day postop.

NURSING INTERVENTIONS:

a. Reduce pain to a level of 4 or less on a 1–10 scale.
b. Explain the at-risk problem and outcome to patient.
c. Explain preventive function of the following activities.
   (1) Turning, coughing, and deep breathing at least every 2 hours.
   (2) Early ambulation.
   (3) Use of deep-breathing device, qlh (incentive spirometer).
d. Explain ways to minimize discomfort during turning and coughing: splinting, analgesics.
e. Offer pain medication 1/2 hour before ambulating.
f. Assist patient to
   (1) TCH q2h × 24 h.
   (2) Ambulate qid starting first postop day.
   (3) Deep breathe qh while awake × 24 h.
g. Assess lung sounds before and after TCH sessions.

• **Whenever possible, nursing actions should be important to the patient and compatible with personal goals and values.** The patient should understand how the nursing actions will result in achievement of the outcome. For example, a man may refuse to do arm and hand exercises because he does not think they are important. If the nursing actions encourage the patient to do activities such as shaving, combing his hair, brushing his teeth, and feeding himself, the arms and hands will still receive the desired exercise. The difference is that the patient values being able to do these self-care activities and can see that they are part of his recovery.

PATIENT TEACHING: AN INTERVENTION STRATEGY

If the nurse assesses a patient and makes a nursing diagnosis with an etiology or risk factors related to a knowledge or performance deficit, a teaching plan will most likely constitute a large portion of the activity in the planning phase of the nursing process. Many plans of care include a teaching component for each outcome as the nurse explains what is to be done and why. Standards by the Joint Commission on the Accreditation of Healthcare Organizations (JCAHO) for hospital accreditation include requirements for the assessment of a patient's learning needs and education about safe and effective use of medications, medical equipment, drug-food interaction, nutrition, modified diets, rehabilitation techniques, community resources, personal hygiene and grooming, and patients' responsibility for continuing health care needs for themselves or family members. Unrealistic fears of a medical procedure and incorrectly taking prescribed

medications are examples of problems that could be caused by erroneous information. Patients with newly diagnosed medical problems frequently are confronted with knowledge deficits concerning the implications of their medical diagnosis and the effect it may have on their life-style. Patients taking on new roles, such as parenting, frequently are concerned about their lack of knowledge and skill in newborn care. Prenatal classes will anticipate these learning needs and identify specific areas of newborn care that prospective parents would like to discuss in class. Nursing follow-through in the hospital, after delivery, builds on this information and gives the parents actual practice in caring for their newborn. Similarly, preoperative and postoperative teaching is based on a nursing diagnosis of inadequate knowledge of the surgical experience, complications, and preventive measures. Preoperative teaching also is based on research indicating that an educated patient, knowing what will happen during a procedure, will often experience less pain and anxiety than will an unprepared patient. The nursing diagnosis again would relate to inadequate or incorrect information about a particular procedure or surgery.

In applying the nursing process to the formulation of a teaching plan, the nurse follows a logical sequence of problem solving. First, the knowledge deficit is identified, based on data obtained during the assessment phase of the nursing process. A learning outcome is then chosen. Next, a plan is developed to teach the skill or information to the patient and family, as appropriate.

For example:

1. NURSING DIAGNOSIS: Knowledge and skill deficit in taking newborn rectal temperature related to first-time parenting.
   [This diagnosis might be written in an alternative form identifying inadequate knowledge and skill as the cause of a potential problem; "High risk for altered health maintenance related to lack of knowledge and skill in newborn temperature assessment."]
   OUTCOME: Take an accurate rectal temperature on her newborn before discharge on 3/5.
   NURSING INTERVENTIONS: (Teaching Plan):
   1. Discuss when to take baby's temperature; signs and symptoms indicating illness.
   2. Demonstrate how to take rectal temperatures on newborns, 3/4.
   3. Explain safety precautions and when to notify physician for fevers, 3/4.
   4. Provide reinforced practice in taking her newborn's temperature, 3/4.

2. NURSING DIAGNOSIS: Knowledge and skill deficit in taking medications related to forgetting and not reading directions.
   [This diagnosis might be written in an alternative form identifying the problem as caused by inadequate knowledge; "High risk for injury related to lack of knowledge of medications and administration."]
   OUTCOME: Demonstrate correct self-administration of medication by 11/3.

NURSING INTERVENTIONS:
1. Check that patient can read all labels on medications, 11/1.
2. Discuss with the patient how to safely take each medication (drug, dose, time, route), 11/1.
3. Provide a clear set of directions in written form regarding medications, 11/1.
4. Supervise patient in hospital with self-administration of prescribed medications, 11/1, 11/2.

When patients and families learn specific motor skills, the outcome selected has a very direct relationship to the diagnosed knowledge or performance deficit. The teaching plan and eventually the evaluation of the patient's ability to perform the skill are usually equally specific. When teaching motor skills, follow the steps of the nursing process:

1. Assess current knowledge and skill ability (ASSESS).
2. Identify knowledge deficits (MAKE NURSING DIAGNOSIS).
   —Inadequate skill in performance of . . .
   —Knowledge deficit in the area of . . .
   —High risk for (specify problem) related to lack of knowledge and/or skill in the area of . . .
3. Identify the specific behavior the patient will perform based on the diagnosed learning need (IDENTIFY OUTCOMES).
4. Decide exactly what to teach and what methods to use, such as demonstration, video, explanation, and written instructions (PLANNING INTERVENTIONS).
5. Teach the specific behavior to the patient (IMPLEMENT).
6. Evaluate the patient's ability to perform the specific behavior (EVALUATE).

Evaluating patient learning may be difficult if observable behaviors are not identified as outcomes. When a patient is developing an understanding of broader concepts or improving cognitive skills, the nurse's teaching plan cannot focus on one specific behavior as evidence of this broader understanding. For example, if the diagnosis relates to inadequate knowledge of infant care, an outcome dealing with the isolated behavior of diapering does not provide support for the assumption that the parent is competent in infant care. In this case, the method the nurse may use is the identification of one long-term learning outcome and then the identification of several subsequent intermediate outcomes that build toward the long-term outcome. The long-term outcome may be more difficult to state in behavioral terms. The examples of intermediate outcomes should be stated as observable or measurable behaviors. The teaching plan is then directed at the discharge outcome by achieving the intermediate outcomes.

Example 1:
NURSING DIAGNOSIS: Knowledge and skill deficit of newborn care related to new parent role.
LONG-TERM OUTCOME: Parents will safely care for newborn by time of discharge from hospital on 11/3.
INTERMEDIATE OUTCOME:
1. Demonstrate bathing their newborn, 11/2.
2. Safely take a rectal temperature on newborn, 11/2.
3. Demonstrate cord care for umbilical stump, 11/2.
4. Breast-feeding: 10–15 minutes per breast q2–5h, by 11/3.
5. Transport newborn home from hospital in infant car seat, 11/3.

TEACHING PLAN: Nursing Interventions
1. Assess readiness for learning infant care (comfort level, fatigue, personal priority needs).
2. Discuss various aspects of infant care: feeding, hygiene, safety, growth and development, behavior.
3. Demonstrate specific infant care skills and provide practice for parents with positive reinforcement.
4. Assist in initiation of breast-feeding and provide specific information on the skill.
5. Provide resources for parents after discharge (people to call when questions or problems arise).
6. Follow-up phone call to answer questions 2–3 days after discharge.

Example 2:
NURSING DIAGNOSIS: High risk for failure in Nursing 101 related to lack of knowledge of the nursing process as evidenced by 2 correct out of 15 points on the unit test.
LONG-TERM OUTCOME: Student will pass Nursing 101 with a grade of "C" or better by the end of the course.
INTERMEDIATE OUTCOMES:
1. Identify six phases of the nursing process, 3/1.
2. Explain nursing diagnosis and how it differs from medical diagnosis, 3/5.
3. Write three nursing diagnoses from a data base, 3/10.
4. Write three nursing outcomes showing observable patient behavior and criteria of performance, 3/20.
5. Write three sets of nursing interventions to help a patient achieve three different outcomes by 4/1.
6. Evaluate achievement of outcomes and review care plan by 4/10.

TEACHING PLAN: Nursing Interventions
1. Assess readiness to learn, strengths and interfering factors.
2. Discuss ways to reduce or eliminate factors interfering with learning.
3. Discuss rationale for using the nursing process.
4. Explain briefly the relationship between the nursing process, patient care, and passing Nursing 101.

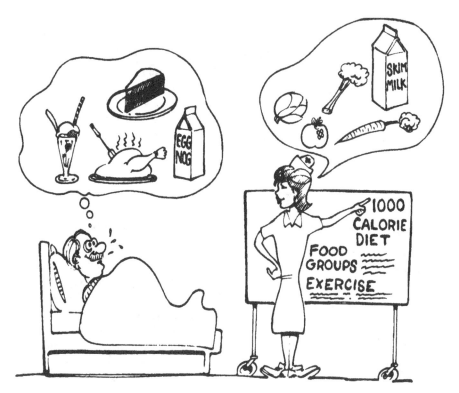

FIGURE 5-2. A good teaching plan does not always guarantee that patient learning will occur.

5. Assign readings on nursing process.
6. Demonstrate application of nursing process on a hypothetical patient's data base.
7. Use practice exercises for writing nursing diagnoses, outcomes, and planning actions.
8. Written student assignment: Develop a care plan on four assigned hospital patients showing assessment, diagnosis, outcome identification, planning, implementation, and evaluation.
9. Review and critique other students' care plans.

There are several things to consider when developing a teaching plan. Learning is enhanced by using principles of teaching-learning. It is especially important to assess the patient's readiness to learn. An illness, medical problem, or treatment may greatly interfere with learning, particularly in the acute phase of an illness. Medications, fatigue, anxiety, pain, or hunger may all block effective learning. Grief over an unexpected medical diagnosis, life-style changes, body changes, or prognosis often will delay the desire for learning by the patient.

For example, the patient who finally begins to look at her colostomy stoma and asks some questions about it may be ready to listen to some information, while a few days ago she was unwilling to even acknowledge the presence of the colostomy as part of her body. Teaching should be delayed until some of these obstacles have been lessened or eliminated. The nurse assesses the patient's current knowledge and skills, building on this base. Begin at the level of patient and family understanding, using language understandable to them. Individualizing the teaching approach may also lead to improved learning.

Common Components of a Teaching Plan	Rationale and Scientific Principles
1. Setting a learning outcome with the patient.	1. Clarification of desired learning outcomes will guide teaching methods and may serve as a motivating function for the learner.
2. Assessing patient's readiness to learn. a. motivation: recognizes knowledge deficit b. illness/medical problem c. medication/pain d. level of consciousness e. anxiety level f. fatigue	2. A person learns more effectively when the learning experience has personal relevance. A person learns more effectively when a need to learn is perceived. Unmet physical or psychosocial needs such as anxiety, pain, and fatigue have a negative effect on attention, retention, and ability to learn.
3. Assess patient's current knowledge and motor skill ability. 4. Begin teaching at the patient's current level of understanding or skill performance.	3, 4. Teaching that moves from simple to complex helps ensure understanding. *Simple* and *complex* are relative terms and have meaning only in relationship to the learner's current level of understanding or performance.
5. Provide the patient with an opportunity to practice motor skills after a demonstration. 6. Reinforce patient's efforts to learn whenever possible.	5, 6. An active learner learns and retains more than does a passive learner. Practice with feedback and positive reinforcement leads to improved performance and continuance of reinforced behavior.

A nurse promotes readiness to learn . . .

I was working in the obstetrical unit of a university hospital. A baby had been born a few days before with a cleft lip and palate. The mother had refused to see or hold the baby since delivery. She stayed in her room, cried frequently, and slept off and on during the day. The staff was getting quite irritated with her since the baby was healthy in every other way and she was supposed to take the baby home the next day. She had refused the information from the doctor on cleft lip and palate. We had delayed all efforts at teaching infant care based on her refusal to do anything with the baby. She was not ready to learn, but the reality of the hospital setting said she would be discharged with that baby the next day, ready or not. The problems of dysfunctional grieving, potential for altered parenting, and even potential for physical harm to the baby were all running through my mind in addition to the knowledge and skill deficit problem. I went in the room, and she pulled the covers over her head and said, "Go away." "Great start," I thought. "This is going to be a terrific shift!" As I sat down in a chair next to her, I was desperately trying to think of what to do. As honestly as I could, I shared my concerns and frustrations as the nurse for her and her baby. I also wanted her to know I wasn't condemning her or telling her she shouldn't feel the way she felt. "I'm so sorry about your baby, and I know you're very upset. You and the baby are supposed to go home tomorrow, and I'm worried because I don't feel like you are ready." I told her what kind of teaching and hands-on care most new mothers are given in the hospital and how they often are still apprehensive about going home. I told her I didn't know how she was feeling or even if she was willing to care for the baby at home. "Your baby is eating very well, acting like all the other babies, crying, sleeping, stooling, and voiding." I was trying to point out what was normal about her baby. After a few moments of silence, I asked the new mother if I could feed her baby in her room because the baby was acting hungry when I left the nursery. The mother agreed, and I held and fed the baby. As I was doing this, she reached out and touched the baby's feet and hands and commented on how perfectly they were formed. As I was leaving the room with the baby after the feeding, she asked me to bring her the information on the cleft lip and palate that the doctor said he would leave at the nurse's station.

CLASSIFICATION OF NURSING INTERVENTIONS

As was discussed in Chapter 4, a research team from the University of Iowa has developed and revised a classification system for nursing interventions. There

are a total of 433 interventions. Interventions initially are divided into six domains:

- *Physiological: Basic.* Care that supports physical functioning
- *Physiological: Complex.* Care that supports homeostatic regulation
- *Behavior:* Care that supports psychological functioning and life-style changes
- *Safety:* Care that supports protection against harm
- *Family:* Care that supports the family unit
- *Health Care System:* Care that supports the effective use of available health care systems

Within each of these six domains there are subdivisions of broad intervention categories. For example, Elimination Management, Activity/Exercise Management, and Physical Comfort Promotion are listed as subdivisions under the domain of Basic Physiological Care. Under each of these broad categories of interventions are lists of specific interventions. Each specific intervention has a label, a definition, and a list of activities for the nurse to carry out with the patient and family in implementing that intervention. The activities listed under each specific intervention are to be selected and individualized on the basis of the nurse's assessment of each patient and family. The specific intervention labels are cross-referenced to the NANDA nursing diagnoses to help nurses base interventions on the patient problem that is identified. The nursing diagnosis of *Pain* is continued with an example of the broad category level of interventions called *Physical Comfort Promotion* in Table 5-1. This is followed by a further breakdown into the more specific intervention label *Pain Management* in Table 5-2.

CRITICAL THINKING FOR PLANNING

As nurses select interventions during the planning phase of the nursing process, they use creativity, knowledge, clinical experience, and patient preferences to adapt and individualize standardized plans of care. The interventions that are chosen are known to have a direct effect on either the problem in the nursing diagnosis or the etiologies of that problem. That is why they are chosen: to reduce, eliminate, or prevent the problem or its cause. This is critical thinking. It is purposeful, creative, reflective reasoning that focuses on deciding what to do to improve the patient's current situation.

Critical thinkers understand the casual relationship between certain interventions and outcomes. They know which interventions have the highest probability of success based on knowledge of anatomy, physiology, nursing, and other sciences and also on clinical experience with patients with similar health problems. Critical thinkers can offer the patient and family more choices and flexibility because they know more options. They understand the principles behind

TABLE 5-1   INTERVENTIONS FOR PHYSICAL COMFORT PROMOTION

DEFINITION: Interventions to promote comfort by using physical techniques

Intervention	*Definition*
Acupressure	Application of firm sustained pressure to special points on the body to decrease pain, produce relaxation, and prevent or reduce nausea
Cutaneous Stimulation	Stimulation of the skin and underlying tissues for the purpose of decreasing undesirable signs and symptoms such as pain, muscle spasms, and inflammation
Environmental Management: Comfort	Manipulation of the patient's surroundings for therapeutic benefit
Heat/Cold Application	Stimulation of the skin and underlying tissues with heat or cold for the purpose of decreasing pain, muscle spasms, or inflammation
Pain Management	Alleviation of pain or a reduction in pain to a level of comfort that is acceptable to the patient (see Table 5-2 for specific activities nurses do to implement this intervention)
Progressive Muscle Relaxation	Facilitating the tensing and releasing of successive muscle groups while attending to the resulting differences in sensation
Simple Massage	Stimulation of the skin and underlying tissues with varying degrees of hand pressure to decrease pain, produce relaxation, and/or improve circulation
Therapeutic Touch	Directing one's own interpersonal energy to flow through the hands to help or heal another person
Transcutaneous Electrical Nerve Stimulation (TENS)	Stimulation of skin and underlying tissues with controlled, low-voltage electrical vibrations via electrodes

Source: Adapted from McCloskey, J., and Bulechek, G. (1996), *Nursing Interventions Classification (NIC)*, 2nd edition. St. Louis, Mosby. Used by permission.

their choices, and this frees them to be creative, to adapt interventions to each unique patient rather than performing routine interventions in the standard way. They view the problem, outcome, and interventions as a whole and include a greater variety of interventions to eliminate not only the problem but the causes of the problem.

Based on patient needs and requests, a critically thinking nurse will reason, "Why not let them do it their way?" or "What if we combine this piece and your piece and do it this way?" The nurse always considers safety as the underlying

TABLE 5-2.   INTERVENTION: PAIN MANAGEMENT

DEFINITION: Alleviation of pain or a reduction in pain to a level of comfort that is acceptable to the patient

Activities nurses use to implement the above intervention:
- Perform a comprehensive assessment of pain to include location, characteristics, onset/duration, frequency, quality, intensity or severity, and precipitating factors
- Observe for nonverbal cues of discomfort, especially in those unable to communicate effectively
- Ensure that the patient receives appropriate analgesic care
- Use therapeutic communication strategies to acknowledge the pain experience and convey acceptance of the patient's response to pain
- Consider cultural influences on pain response
- Determine the impact of the pain experience on quality of life (e.g., sleep, appetite, activity, cognition, mood, relationships, performance of job, and role responsibilities)
- Evaluate past experiences with pain to include individual or family history of chronic pain, or resulting disability as appropriate
- Evaluate with the patient and the health care team the effectiveness of pain control measures that have been used
- Help patient and family seek and provide support
- Use a developmentally appropriate assessment method that allows for monitoring of change in pain and that will assist in identifying actual and potential precipitating factors (e.g., flow sheet and daily diary)
- Determine the needed frequency of making an assessment of patient comfort and implement monitoring plan
- Provide information about the pain, such as causes of the pain, how long it will last, and anticipated discomfort from procedures
- Control environmental factors that may influence the patient's response to discomfort (e.g., room temperature, lighting, and noise)
- Reduce or eliminate factors that precipitate or increase the pain experience (e.g., fear, fatigue, monotony, and lack of knowledge)
- Consider the patient's willingness to participate, ability to participate, preference, support of significant others for method, and contraindications when selecting a pain relief strategy
- Select and implement a variety of measures (e.g., pharmacological, nonpharmacological, and interpersonal) to facilitate pain relief as appropriate
- Consider type and source of pain when selecting pain relief strategy
- Encourage patient to monitor own pain and intervene appropriately
- Teach the use of nonpharmacological techniques (e.g., biofeedback, TENS, hypnosis, relaxation, guided imagery, music therapy, distraction, play therapy, activity therapy, acupressure, hot/cold applications, and massage)

before, after, and, if possible, during painful activities; before pain occurs
or increases; and along with other pain relief measures
- Collaborate with the patient, significant others, and other health
  professionals to select and implement nonpharmacological pain relief
  measures as appropriate
- Provide optimal pain relief with prescribed analgesics
- Implement the use of patient-controlled analgesia (PCA) if appropriate
- Use pain control measures before pain becomes severe
- Medicate before an activity to increase participation, but evaluate the
  hazards of sedation
- Ensure pretreatment analgesia and/or nonpharmacological strategies before
  painful procedures
- Verify level of discomfort with patient, note changes in the medical record,
  and inform other health professionals working with the patient
- Evaluate the effectiveness of the pain control measures used through
  ongoing assessment of the pain experience
- Institute and modify pain control measures on the basis of the patient's
  response
- Promote adequate rest/sleep to facilitate pain relief
- Encourage the patient to discuss the pain experience as appropriate
- Notify physician if measures are unsuccessful or if current complaint
  represents a significant change from patient's past experience of pain
- Inform other health care professionals/family members of
  nonpharmacological strategies being used by the patient to encourage
  preventive approaches to pain management
- Use a multidisciplinary approach to pain management when appropriate
- Consider referrals for patient, family, and significant others to support
  groups and other resources, as appropriate
- Provide accurate information to promote family's knowledge of and
  response to the pain experience
- Incorporate the family in the pain relief modality if possible
- Monitor patient satisfaction with pain management at specific intervals

Source: McCloskey, J., and Bulechek, G. (1996), *Nursing Interventions Classification (NIC)*, 2nd
edition. St. Louis, Mosby. Used by permission.

constant. As long as the intervention is safe or can be made safe, why not? For
example, in some cultures after childbirth, burial of the placenta in a specific
area related to the home of the woman is considered important for the health and
well-being of the child. Can the nurse be part of the solution, or will the nurse
be part of the problem? Should the nurse say, "A placenta is a hazardous waste
and must be disposed of by the hospital. This is mandated by infection control"
or "Tell me about this tradition, about the meaning and what you plan to do with
the placenta. Let me make some calls and see how we can accommodate you"?

Prompts for Critical Thinking during Planning

- Are all interventions safe and consistent with the plan of care?
- Will the interventions selected result in achieving the desired outcome? How do you know?
- What is your reason for selecting this intervention instead of another one? Any biases?
- What are the most important interventions (priorities) from the patient's point of view? Family's? Health professionals'?
- Are the interventions culturally sensitive? Age-appropriate?
- Does the plan build on patient/family strengths and resources and minimize deficits?
- Are the interventions acceptable to the patient? Family?
- Do you need to include other disciplines or ideas from more expert nurses in your plan?
- Are you combining a variety of approaches (at least three) to reduce or eliminate the problem or its cause (for example, combine assessment, teaching, nutrition, oxygenation, and hydration interventions in addition to analgesics when treating pain from surgery, thus reducing the pain directly and helping the incision heal)?
- What alternative, complementary interventions can be used?
- Are the interventions clear? Are there criteria for frequency, timing and duration, or level of the intervention to guide others?

CULTURALLY COMPETENT NURSING CARE DURING PLANNING

Plans that blend Western medicine with cultural values, beliefs, and practices increase adherence and satisfaction with the treatment plan. It is not just a nice thing to do; it is clinically essential if we want to avoid frightening, alienating, and offending patients and families of other cultures. A nurse needs to be open and flexible, using sound principles from the physical and social sciences to guide practice. Principles give the nurse flexibility. A procedure can be done this way or that way or even this other way; all these options maintain safety and achieve the same eventual end. One way is my way, one way is your way, and the third is a blending with which we both feel comfortable. Is there more than one safe and effective way of getting from the problem to its resolution? Creativity and a sound scientific rationale are the basis for your actions.

The American Nurses Association's *Standards of Clinical Nursing Practice* (1998) states that "the plan is individualized to the patient (e.g., culturally sensitive)." To individualize a plan of care, the nurse considers many facets of a patient: physical, psychological, and sociocultural. This is done most effectively by involving people in their own care. The nurse is creative in developing a plan that combines the patient's cultural view of health and health care delivery with

the Western biomedical framework. The nurse talks with patients and asks how this problem might be treated within their culture or under the care of a traditional healer. What do they miss in this setting related to their treatment and care?

Consider the complexity of the health care reimbursement system and realize that families from other cultures may need additional help and guidance to find and use financial resources.

PLANNING

Finding the "Happy" Medium

Setting desired outcomes and the appropriate priorities in order to achieve those outcomes is what planning is all about. Making a plan to reach your desired outcomes that the patient, the family, and the health professional can all agree on is what planning is all about. It was an evening shift when I was called into the ICU. The RN reported that the patient had a dangerously low hematocrit of barely 12 and was in great need of surgery. One problem—he was a Jehovah's Witness. The surgeons felt strongly that the highest priority was the surgery and a blood transfusion. The patient viewed the priorities of the situation from a much different vantage point. His religious convictions allowed him to agree with the need for surgery but required him to refuse the transfusions. The surgeons and the patient were at an impasse. A creative plan of care for this patient was needed. Gathering the facts from both the patient and physician revealed that delaying the surgery to allow the hematocrit to increase naturally was acceptable to both the surgeon and the patient. The patient began on blood expanders. He also agreed to be ventilated and chemically paralyzed to lower his metabolism. The patient was watched carefully until the hematocrit was sufficient for surgery. The surgery was successful without the need for blood, meeting the patient's physical and religious needs without compromising the surgeon's safety standards for medical practice.

R. Peterson, RN, MSN

FIGURE 5-3.

Prompts for Culturally Competent Nursing Care during Planning

- Consider the cultural role of family members and significant others in the plan. What role do they expect to play?

- Provide for the comfort needs of the family members or significant others if their role is to "care for" the sick member.
- Provide opportunities for family or significant others' involvement in care and decision making if this is a cultural expectation.
- Include the patient and family or significant others in plan development to help you include their cultural needs.
- Consider cultural preferences related to diet, food temperatures, clothing, personal hygiene, and grooming needs.
- Adapt the plan on the clinical pathway for patients from other cultures. Remember that most clinical pathways have a Western medicine, white, Anglo-European cultural orientation.
- Develop resources with information on high frequency cultures in your clinical setting.
- Develop clinical pathways that include cultural cues or adaptations for a specific culture.

PLANNING: THE MANAGED CARE ENVIRONMENT

In today's health care environment a tool called a critical pathway has evolved. The pathway may be thought of as a kind of grid with care defined by time periods. This tool specifies which nursing interventions to implement and when to do them for all patients in a particular DRG or with a particular disease state or surgical procedure. Both the critical nursing and the medical interventions usually are included in the critical pathway tool.

In most institutions multidisciplinary teams of health care providers develop critical pathways. A nurse case manager is often the person charged with leading the design team for critical pathways. Because of their clinical expertise, they know all the caregivers who are involved in the care of a certain type of patient. For a patient having total knee replacement surgery, it is essential to involve social workers, physical therapists, home health nurses, pharmacists, operating room (OR) nurses, and nurse educators as well as orthopedic staff nurses and physicians. Many critical pathways begin in an outpatient setting and outline all the care the patient is to receive throughout hospitalization and recovery. Critical pathways are designed to include the most effective interventions to help patients meet identified outcomes. For example, on the day of surgery the critical pathway may direct the nurse to have the patient stand at the bedside that evening. The next day the critical pathway would direct the nurse to ambulate the patient in the hall tid. All these interventions would be aimed at meeting the discharge outcome "Ambulates unassisted with no dizziness by discharge."

The interventions on the critical pathway serve as minimum standards of practice. They define the process (actions) most likely to yield the desired outcomes. Critical pathways and the defined interventions are designed to serve as guidelines for caring for approximately 75% of patients with a particular DRG,

condition, or surgical procedure. However, each individual patient will need the nurse to individualize these standard interventions for maximum effectiveness. Some interventions may need to be modified, some may need to be added, and some may be inappropriate for a particular patient. The time line may need to be altered for an individual patient who is progressing ahead of or behind the expected course.

There are two goals of critical pathways: First, they are designed to provide quality care. As nurses follow the plan of care on a critical pathway, they are quickly able to identify when a patient is not meeting the desired clinical outcomes. The interventions are then modified, and the patient is assessed frequently to assure that the outcomes are being met. The second goal—cost effectiveness—is met because the interventions on a pathway have been evaluated and selected carefully as those that will meet the clinical outcomes for the lowest cost.

Pathways that have been designed by multidisciplinary teams result in a multidisciplinary plan of care. Both managed care companies and the organization that accredits hospitals (JCAHO) have been supportive of the development of critical pathways, recognizing that both quality of care and cost-effectiveness requirements are being met.

See Table 6-1 (p. 170f) for an example of a critical pathway for a patient having total knee replacement therapy surgery. The staff members at this institution document on the critical pathway by using a system called charting by exception. A check mark (✓) on the pathway indicates that the intervention or outcome was within the parameters specified on the pathway. An asterisk (*) indicates that a change from the pathway has occurred and that a narrative-style progress note will be found.

SUMMARY

Nursing interventions are the specific activities the nurse plans and implements to help the patient achieve desired outcomes. There are four broad categories of nursing interventions, and the plan of care often incorporates actions from several of those groups: environmental management, physician-ordered and -initiated interventions, physician-ordered and nurse-initiated interventions, and nurse-ordered and initiated interventions. The last group of interventions is solely within the realm of nursing practice and includes health teaching, health promotion, counseling, and referral; specific nursing treatments; assisting with activities of daily living (ADLs); assessment of patient status, progress, and response; assistance with problem solving; discharge planning; maximizing nutrition; and providing encouragement and hope. Nursing interventions deal with the problem and the etiology or risk factors identified in the nursing diagnosis and try to reduce or eliminate them. If that is not possible, interventions are aimed at lessening the problematic signs and symptoms to help the patient

and family cope with the problem. Nursing interventions are safe for the patient, specific, congruent with the plans of other health care professionals, and realistic for the patient, the nurse, and the health care setting.

CASE STUDY: PLANNING

The case study of Mrs. Wiley is continued from Chapter 4 to identify a plan of care.

#1 PLANNING
PREOPERATIVE ORTHOPEDIC SURGERY CLINIC

Mrs. Wiley: Plan of care is designed by the nurse in the orthopedic clinic.

Nursing Diagnoses	Clinical Outcomes	Interventions	Rationale
Knowledge deficit: strengthening exercises, crutch walking, pain management after surgery, use of incentive spirometer, preoperative preparation for surgery	Verbalize/demonstrate: strengthening exercises, anticipated length of stay, what to expect during hospitalization, understanding of pain management and pain rating scale, use of incentive spirometer, crutch walking	Teach patient and family: 1. Pain management after surgery (PCA) 2. Preoperative routines/instructions 3. Offer advance directives 4. Equipment: continuous passive motion machine 5. Refer to home health nursing for home assessment 6. Refer to physical therapy to teach crutch walking	1. Teaching the patient and family before they are in the stressful situation of surgery will enhance learning. 2. As above. 3. Per hospital policy, all patients are offered this information. 4. See (1) above. 5. Identify potential hazards to safety. 6. Easier to learn the skills before surgery.

Nursing Diagnoses	Clinical Outcomes	Interventions	Rationale
Husband: risk for injury related to absence of care provider	Husband will remain injury-free during absence and recovery of primary caregiver (Mrs. Wiley).	1. Discuss/clarify needs with patient and husband 2. Document and communicate needs to home health nurse.	1. Determine whether the family has plans for meeting needs. 2. Plan for additional home health care for both Mr. and Mrs. Wiley on a temporary basis after surgery.
Chronic pain related to degeneration of knee joint	Patient will state that pain is controlled at 4 or less on activity or less than 2 at rest until the time of surgery.	1. Assess what Mrs. Wiley is taking, how frequently, and level of relief. 2. Communicate pain need to physician. 3. Instruct patient about new medication. 4. Teach noninvasive pain control: application of cold, distraction, relaxation tapes.	1. Clarify understanding of what medication is not effective. 2. May need to adjust medications to make patient comfortable in the 2 weeks before surgery and put the patient in the best possible condition for surgery. 3. Promote self-care and autonomy. 4. Supplement medication with noninvasive pain control measures to maximize relief.

#2 PLANNING
FIRST DAY SURGERY CENTER: 6 A.M.

Patients are admitted to the first day surgery center the morning of surgery for their scheduled procedures and are transferred to the inpatient unit after surgery.

Mrs. Wiley: Plan of care is designed by the nurse at the time of admission, 6 A.M. day of surgery.

Nursing Diagnoses	Clinical Outcomes	Interventions	Rationale
Fear of reduced mobility related to outcome of surgery	Patient will report reduced fear levels before leaving preop prep area.	1. Encourage patient to verbalize and clarify fears. 2. Have family member/nurse remain with patient until patient goes to OR. 3. Share experience of typical patient with this surgery and outcomes of less pain and more mobility. 4. Offer comfort measures: warm blanket, pillows.	1. Identifying the fear and naming it enable patient to cope more effectively. 2. Fears can become exaggerated when patient is alone without social support. 3. Without giving false reassurance, nurse can say, "It has been my experience that most patients with this type of surgery feel great pain relief and improved mobility within a very short time." 4. Pain/discomfort enhances fear.
Risk for injury (Mrs. Wiley) related to lack of experience with crutch walking	Patient will be injury-free during hospitalization and home recovery.	1. Communicate to nurse on postop unit in writing and in care plan. 2. Teach safe crutch walking on flat surface and on stairs before discharge.	1. Document this safety need to assure that it does not get lost during multiple shift changes. 2. Increase patient safety and mobility.
Anxiety (patient and family members) related to surgical experience	Patient and family will demonstrate reduced anxiety within 6 hours, as evidenced by: patient or family will state relief at outcomes of surgery.	1. Orient family members to waiting area, cafeteria. 2. Give written phone numbers of postoperative unit, assigned postoperative room.	1. Reduces strangeness of environment. 2. Creates tangible links to family member.

Nursing Diagnoses	Clinical Outcomes	Interventions	Rationale
		3. Tell them how, where, and when they will obtain information.	3. Reduces uncertainty.
		4. Offer beverages and/or directions to cafeteria.	4. Comfort measures to create caring environment.

#3 PLANNING
POSTOPERATIVE ORTHOPEDIC PATIENT CARE UNIT

Mrs. Wiley: Plan of care is designed by the nurse during the first hours after surgery.

Nursing Diagnoses	Clinical Outcomes	Interventions	Rationale
Acute pain related to joint replacement surgery, movement, and physical therapy	Pain will remain at 3 or less throughout hospitalization.	1. Assess pain at least every 2 hours.	1. Pain med may need to be adjusted. Healing and mobility are impeded by pain.
		2. Reinforce teaching on PCA pump.	2. Patient may not understand or hesitate to use. Emphasize early intervention at low pain levels.
		3. Record pain intensity, intervention, and response.	3. Document individual response and identify what is successful.
		4. Review dose and meds for possible changes.	4. May consider adding NSAID, if ordered, to opioid to enhance relief.
		5. Teach relaxation techniques.	5. Complementary non-pharmacological intervention.
		6. Encourage patient to use PCA before PT.	6. Enhance ability to participate in therapy.

Nursing Diagnoses	Clinical Outcomes	Interventions	Rationale
Risk for caregiver role strain (upon discharge) related to dependency of frail spouse and surgery of caregiver	Caregiver and husband will identify needs at home and plan for assistance during care planning conference.	1. As part of discharge plan, discuss with patient, husband, and family who does what tasks in household. 2. Identify tasks Mrs. Wiley will be unable to complete for a time. 3. Clarify Mrs. Wiley's needs for rest and activity during rehab. 4. Problem solve additional sources of aid. 5. Communicate to the home health agency selected by Mr. and Mrs. Wiley.	1. Gain perceptions of family members and enlist their support. 2. Anticipatory discharge planning. 3. Mrs. Wiley will heal faster with adequate rest and nutrition. 4. Determine what resources the family has and what assistance the Wileys are willing to accept. 5. Continuity of care for patient and family.
Impaired physical mobility, level 2*, related to knee replacement surgery	Patient will manage independent ambulation with crutches by discharge.	1. Teach use of trapeze to assist movement. 2. Teach placement of crutches to facilitate getting out of bed, out of chair, up from toilet. 3. Teach upper-arm resistance exercises with 2- to 5-lb weight.	1. Facilitate movement in bed and weight shifting to reduce pressure areas. 2. Enhance safety and mobility. 3. Strengthen upper arms and increase circulation.
Risk for injury (Mrs. Wiley) related to lack of experience with crutch walking	Patient will remain free of falls during hospitalization and home recovery.	1. Premedicate 1 hour before physical therapy. 2. Physical therapist to instruct in crutch walking and transfers. 3. Supervised 2/day physical therapy while in hospital.	1. Enhance ability to participate in physical therapy. 2. Repeated instructions and practice to accomplish new skill. 3. Maximize strength and skill.

Nursing Diagnoses	Clinical Outcomes	Interventions	Rationale
		4. Evaluate for at-home physical therapy upon discharge.	4. With limited assistance at home, Mrs. Wiley needs to be confident in her ability and safe in home environment.

* Requires help from another person for assistance, supervision, or teaching.

#4 PLANNING
HOME HEALTH CARE AGENCY

Mrs. Wiley: Plan of care is designed by the nurse at the time of the home health visit.

Nursing Diagnoses	Clinical Outcomes	Interventions	Rationale
Knowledge/ skill deficit: Signs/ symptoms to report to MD; aseptic technique; self-admin-istered medication, purpose, schedule; wound care; pain man-agement techniques	Reports elevated temperature/ chills to MD within 2 hours. Attains healing of wound without compli-cations within 14 days. Demonstrates aseptic technique during wound care by second visit.	1. Teach S/S of infection to report to MD. 2. Teach aseptic technique for dressing changes. 3. Change dressing at incision site and instruct patient in assessment and process.	1. Patient is prone to infection due to age, surgical wound, and immobility. Recogni-nition of S/S could enable early treatment. 2. Prevention of infection. 3. Promote healing and permit assessment.
Acute pain related to joint re-placement surgery, physical therapy, and movement	Maintains pain at 2 or less during week 1 at home.	1. Teach pain man-agement techniques: relaxation, medication, cold application. 2. Alternate OTC meds and Tylenol #3. 3. Medicate 1 hour before PT.	1. Methods to enhance pain relief to use alone or in combi-nation with medication. 2. Enhance efficacy of narcotic. 3. Enhance ability to participate in PT.

Nursing Diagnoses	Clinical Outcomes	Interventions	Rationale
Risk for injury (Mrs. Wiley) related to lack of experience with crutch walking	Remains free of falls at home.	1. Reinforce PT exercises. 2. Teach resistance exercises for upper-body strength, using soup cans for weights. 3. Assess home for hazards with each visit: wet floors, cluttered steps, unsafe basement steps, home entrances. Suggest night-lights, steps, railings, grab bars. 4. Discuss winter weather precautions.	1. Increase patient's self-confidence. 2. Strengthen upper arms to support crutch walking. 3. Movement of furniture/objects could present safety hazard for patient. 4. Ice and snow are a special hazard to elderly patients at risk for falls.

CHAPTER 6

Implementation

STANDARD V. IMPLEMENTATION

The Nurse Implements the Interventions Identified in the Plan of Care.

Reprinted with permission from American Nurses Association, *Standards of Clinical Nursing Practice*, 2nd edition, © 1998 American Nurses Publishing, American Nurses Foundation/American Nurses Association, Washington, D.C.

Like the other steps in the nursing process, the implementation phase consists of several activities: validating the care plan, writing the care plan, giving and documenting nursing care, and continuing to collect data.

$$\text{Implementing} = \frac{\text{Validating}}{\text{Care Plan}} + \frac{\text{Documenting}}{\text{Care Plan}} + \frac{\text{Giving and}}{\text{Documenting}} + \frac{\text{Continuing}}{\text{Data}}$$
$$\text{Nursing Care} \quad \text{Collection}$$

VALIDATING THE CARE PLAN

When nursing students or inexperienced staff nurses write care plans, it is recommended that they take the proposed care plans to a colleague and request validation. This step does not have to involve a lengthy scheduled consultation but is a very brief time during which nurses seek the opinion of other nurses. It is important that the student seek appropriate sources for validation. For example, the student may ask the clinical instructor or responsible staff nurse to review the care plan. Such qualified sources can evaluate the care plan by using the following questions as guides:

1. Does the plan assure the patient's safety?
2. Is the plan based on sound scientific principles?
3. Is the plan supported by accepted nursing knowledge?
4. Are the nursing diagnoses supported by the data? Are the major defining characteristics present?
5. Do priorities consider patient preferences and physical and psychosocial needs?
6. Do the outcomes relate to the problems identified in the nursing diagnoses?
7. Do the outcomes contain a time and patient behavior for evaluation?
8. Can the planned nursing actions realistically help the patient achieve the intended outcomes?
9. Are the nursing actions arranged in a logical sequence?
10. Is the plan individualized to the needs and capabilities of this particular patient?
11. Is the plan congruent with the standards, protocols, and procedures for the particular health care setting? With the plans of other health care professionals?

Thus, the nurse who provides the validation is reviewing the plan in four major areas:

1. Safety
2. Appropriateness
3. Effectiveness
4. Individualized nursing care

Because of their expertise in nursing care, other nurses are the most frequently used resource for validation. At times, a nurse may wish to utilize another health team member to review some aspect of a nursing care plan. For example, a nurse teaching a diabetic patient about a diabetic exchange diet may wish to have a dietitian validate the food substitutions requested by the patient and family.

Occasionally, a nursing student may select an inappropriate person to validate a care plan. Frequently, nursing assistants are very knowledgeable about a specific type of care, having had several years' experience in a particular clinical area. However, a nursing student should not ask nursing assistants to validate a care plan. Nursing assistants may be a source for data in that they may be able to provide information about routines of the clinical area, but they are not planners of nursing care. This is a function of the professional nurse.

Having reviewed the plan with another nursing professional, the student or nurse may wish to share the completed plan with the patient, who is another possible source for validation. The patient or family can advise the nurse if any aspect of the plan is unacceptable. This gives patients another opportunity to participate in planning their own care. In summary, to validate the plan is to ask another appropriate professional and the patient, if possible, to approve the plan for implementation.

DOCUMENTING THE NURSING CARE PLAN

To retain a nursing care plan for the exclusive use of one nurse is to defeat a primary purpose of care plans. To get the maximum effect, a care plan must get the maximum press.

A nurse may plan a patient care conference as a "press conference" for a completed care plan. At such a meeting the nurse summarizes data, problems, outcomes, and planned actions. The nurse spends most of the time focusing on presenting the care plan to other nurses. At this time the nurse also may gain new information to add to the care plan. This conference may be used as a problem-solving session during which a nurse may request assistance from colleagues to further develop a care plan.

Interdisciplinary care conferences involve various professionals, such as the physician, physical therapist, social worker, dietitian, and chaplain, in addition to the patient's primary nurse. All these professionals work together to develop a plan of care for the patient, focusing on long-term outcomes and interventions. The patient and family participate in this problem-solving group whenever possible.

The change of shift report is another time when the nurse shares concerns about patients, seeks additional data or suggestions from colleagues, identifies problems, sets priorities, identifies intermediate outcomes, and plans interven-

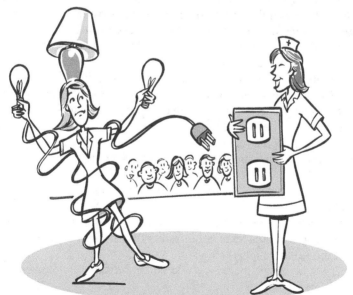

" And now your two favorite nursing instructors will help you understand the nursing diagnosis of 'Powerlessness' by doing a little skit for you"

FIGURE 6-1.   Implementation of a well-developed plan: teaching that comes alive for the learners to promote real understanding.

tions. This process will direct the nurse's activities during the coming 8-hour shift. The nurse can delegate or clarify activities for other health team members so that everyone knows what is important to assess and report and what to do for or with the patient/family over the next few hours.

There are several charting formats, depending on the type of facility in which care is given. All serve as a communication tool.

The charting generally involves continued reporting of data on the patient and the medical and/or nursing diagnoses, an interpretation of those data in relationship to the problem, changes or additions to nursing actions, and evaluation of outcomes after these interventions are implemented.

Other hospitals use a nursing Kardex as a system for organizing care plans. A nursing Kardex is a file that contains the nursing care plans. Each plan is recorded on an oversized index card or a large folded sheet of paper. Kardex forms may include space for medical treatments, diagnostic procedures, and other schedules. Still other institutions have adopted 8 1/2-inch × 11-inch nursing care plan forms, which have the advantage of corresponding to standard chart size.

Some hospitals are using the computer to generate a standardized care plan for a patient with a specific diagnosis. The nurse begins with this care plan and then modifies it to meet the needs of the individual patient. Other health care settings are "filling in the blanks" to individualize a preprinted standard care plan developed by more-expert nurses.

The form of the written care plan may vary from institution to institution, but it should be a useful tool for communication. Most include space for nursing diagnoses, outcomes, nursing interventions, and evaluation in an abbreviated form. A written care plan may be condensed but must convey all the essential information. Often nurses use worksheets to record problems, intermediate outcomes, and interventions that will be accomplished during their 8-hour shift.

This 8-hour plan does not need to be written as a permanent care plan, although the nursing care must be documented in the patient's chart and a report must be given to the next shift of nurses. The written care plan should be used to communicate outcomes achieved by the patient.

The following suggestions will help the nurse write a care plan.

1. Abbreviate whenever possible, using standardized medical or English symbols.
2. Choose key words to communicate ideas; do not write whole sentences.
3. Refer people to procedure books rather than trying to include all the steps for a procedure on a written plan.
4. Category headings should include nursing diagnoses, outcomes, nursing actions, and outcome evaluations.
5. The nursing diagnosis with the related outcomes and nursing actions should appear on the care plan.
6. Include a date for the evaluation of each outcome.
7. All long-term and discharge outcomes should be written. Nursing actions directly related to these outcomes also should be written. If intermediate

outcomes will be evaluated within the nurse's 8-hour shift, it is not necessary to include them on the written form. It is necessary to document the nursing care and the patient outcome that actually occurred.

8. Intermediate outcomes that cannot be met within an 8-hour shift should be written so that other nurses can continue the plan of care.

9. Long-term and discharge outcomes being met by a series of intermediate outcomes belong on the Kardex and/or in the patient's chart. The accompanying actions for intermediate outcomes are included. If the intermediate outcome is to be met during the next few hours by the nurse writing the care plan, the nurse should write the next progressive intermediate outcome and nursing actions.

10. When intermediate outcomes are evaluated, they should be signed and dated by the responsible nurse.

11. All nursing interventions (actions, orders, or whatever term is being used) should be signed by the registered nurse responsible for writing them.

GIVING AND DOCUMENTING NURSING CARE

At last! The nurse now has a plan that will individualize the care given to a patient. Now the nurse is ready to give the care as planned. Even though the nurse has developed an excellent care plan, occasionally (and in the hospital it seems to be the rule), situations occur that interfere with implementing the plan. The patient may be scheduled for emergency surgery. A patient may be in great pain, which alters priorities. Visitors may arrive, and the patient is eager to spend time with them. In each case the nurse may be unable to implement the care plan without making some modifications. There are times when the nurse believes that the performance of certain assessments, treatments, and activities is necessary for the patient's physical safety. Patients, families, and other health care workers may then have to reset their priorities, reschedule, or modify what they were planning. For example, a newborn with an admitting rectal temperature of 96° F is hypothermic, and interventions to stabilize and raise the temperature should be implemented immediately. Any activities with the newborn, such as bathing and removing the baby from the warmer, might worsen the problem or interfere with treatment and should be delayed until the temperature is back in the normal range. The nurse discusses the problem, desired outcome, and interventions with the family and others working with this newborn. The nurse may problem solve with the family at this time to identify alternative ways to meet family needs while still guaranteeing treatment for the hypothermia. For example, parents could keep the baby in their room under the warmer for picture taking and to prevent separation.

Finally, as a last step in implementation, the nurse documents the care given to patients and their response. The nurse is guided by the old maxim "If it is not recorded, it has not been done." If evidence of implementation does not exist in the patient's permanent record, it would seem that the plan has not been

followed and the efforts of the nurse have been wasted. In addition, following the nursing interventions planned by a colleague is a way in which nurses support each other in developing accountability for nursing care. Few nurses would omit giving or documenting a medication ordered by a physician. The implementation of nursing interventions is equally important to the well-being of patients and thus deserves to be treated seriously, respectfully, and with full accountability.

Even the best-laid plans sometimes run amok . . .

I was a nursing instructor working with a young, attractive, single male nursing student on the labor and delivery area. We had discussed how uncomfortable he felt, and he jokingly said his goal for this clinical rotation was to avoid seeing a birth. We laughed, but I said I could accept that as long as he was responsible for the theoretical content and had some experience with the monitors and assessments. His eyes lit up as he scanned the Kardex, and he chose to follow two women in preterm labor where the goal of medical management was to stop their labor. When he began to follow them, both women were experiencing almost no contractions but had fetal and uterine monitors. He was feeling quite smug about his assignment and relieved that it looked like his personal goal was a "given." As he walked past a patient's room on the way to the desk, he heard the patient scream out "Help! Help! The baby's coming!" He confided later that the thought crossed his mind to keep on walking, but he stopped and went in. The woman was in a small panic, and a look under the covers at the bulging perineum confirmed the reason for her distress. Just then the staff nurse with whom the student was working came into the room responding to the call light. "Saved!" he thought as he headed for the door. His nurse told him in no uncertain terms that he was helping her, and within a few minutes they had delivered the baby. I knew nothing of all this, but I ran into him about 15 minutes after the birth and casually asked if he had gotten down for supper yet. "Supper!" he replied. "I just delivered a baby! I may never eat again!"

CONTINUING DATA COLLECTION

Throughout the process of implementation the nurse continues to collect data. As the patient's condition changes, the data base changes, subsequently requiring revising and updating of the care plan. Data gathered while giving nursing care also may be used as evidence for evaluation of outcome achievement, which will be discussed in Chapter 7.

CRITICAL THINKING FOR IMPLEMENTATION

The activities of validating and documenting the plan and actually implementing the plan with the patient while continuing to collect data require the nurse to be a critical thinker. Courage in showing another person your plan and humility in using constructive criticism or seeking out more knowledgeable and experienced nurses are characteristics of critical thinkers. Their reasoning is purposeful: the best intervention given in the most competent and timely manner to each patient. Clear, logical reasoning and assessment skills are needed as care is provided. The expected or the unexpected may occur. Will you recognize the difference? The nurse needs to assess the patient's actual response. Assessing the patient with biased eyes could lead the nurse to falsely think the desired response occurred.

A critically thinking nurse will hold standards of high-quality patient care up against personal feelings when things don't go as well as they might. Extra effort and rethinking the plan with the help of others may be required for the good of the patient. The nurse has "gotta wanta know" why something did not work or why the patient could not or would not participate as expected. Maybe the nurse's knowledge and skills need upgrading. Maybe something was overlooked because of the nurse's biases. Reflective self-examination and application of standards to one's own behavior take courage and integrity. You have your plan, the time is now, your lunch break is coming, and you want to get this done. Whose priorities are at work here? The critical thinker knows. Do you?

Prompts for Critical Thinking during Implementation

- Do you understand the whole plan (not just interventions to carry out)?
- Are you following the plan correctly? Are you timely with your interventions?
- What is the patient's current status? Has it changed? Are the problems still the same?
- How is the patient responding during this intervention? Is the intervention safe? Is it being tolerated?
- Should this intervention be altered to better fit the patient's actual status?
- What is the patient's response after the intervention? Do new interventions need to be added on the basis of this response?
- Who are the "expert" nurses you can go to for help if the patient's responses to your interventions are not what you anticipated?
- Is there a need to alter future interventions in any way? Why and how? Whom do you tell?
- Are there new problems? How do you know? Do you need more data to confirm?

CULTURALLY COMPETENT NURSING CARE DURING IMPLEMENTATION

"The nurse delivers care in a nonjudgmental and nondiscriminatory manner that is sensitive to patient diversity" (ANA, *Standards of Professional Performance*, 1998). Consider verbal and nonverbal cues from the patient and family as you provide care. If it seems that they are upset or concerned about what is being done, stop and clarify. Verbal and nonverbal messages can be easily misunderstood. Remember that direct eye contact from the patient to you may be inappropriate in the patient's culture and the lack of direct eye contact may not be a sign of inattention. Suggest an interpreter during care if needed or have one available by phone. Ask for suggestions from more experienced nurses or from interpreters if the patient and family are responding in unanticipated ways to the delivery of care.

Prompts for Culturally Competent Nursing Care during Implementation

- Have an interpreter present during actual care if there is a language barrier.
- Give the patient privacy from the interpreter during personal care.
- Are there cultural needs for modesty and a same-sex nurse when personal care is provided? This should be considered in making out the nurse's daily patient assignments.
- Have translated materials available before teaching or explaining.
- Use titles and proper names for patients as a sign of respect.
- Be aware of your own verbal and nonverbal communication; identify and eliminate behaviors that can be offensive to the cultures with which you work.
- Avoid technical jargon and slang expressions to promote understanding.
- Touching the head may be disrespectful.
- Cultural practices and traditions are often comforting, so incorporate them into the patient's care as long as they are safe.

IMPLEMENTATION: THE MANAGED CARE ENVIRONMENT

The first step in the implementation phase of the nursing process is validating the care plan. If the nurse is using a critical pathway, a multidisciplinary team has already validated the plan through the process of developing the pathway. The pathway is a tool that represents clinical experts' ideas on what constitutes the best care for a group of average patients admitted with the same DRG, disease condition, or surgical procedure. The pathway reflects a multidisciplinary approach with the actions of all involved health care professionals identified on a time grid.

How a nurse actually works with the patient and family to implement a plan of care changes with technology, the nursing care delivery system, and the work environment. However, regardless of the health care delivery system, the nurse responds to the patient's current status and needs when giving direct care. The nurse directs interventions toward achieving outcomes in all delivery systems. With the use of critical pathways and/or case management, the nurse's role in validating the plan as appropriate for this patient and individualizing care is even more critical. This is the case because the care plan is based not on one individual's particular needs but on the common needs and problems of a large group of patients admitted under the same DRG.

The following questions will help you individualize care when using a critical pathway:

1. Are there clinical outcomes that serve as the goals for each nursing diagnosis you have identified for the patient? The individual patient may have comorbidities (other disease conditions that exist along with the admitting diagnosis) that are not addressed on the critical pathway. Examples of common comorbidities include diabetes, hypertension, asthma, and obesity. Each of these disease states requires that both nursing diagnoses and outcomes be identified. Alcoholism is another frequently seen disease that may result in complications during hospitalization. Some expert nurses who work in chemical dependency centers advise doubling the amount of alcohol a patient reports to get a more accurate measure. Patients who are chemically dependent may have altered reactions to anesthesia and pain management.

2. Are the nursing interventions on the critical pathway appropriate for this patient? The nurse will add interventions to a critical pathway to address comorbidities. For example, patients who are having surgery and have insulin-dependent diabetes require special assessments and care. Some institutions may use more than one critical pathway at the same time. One pathway would be primary. Perhaps the patient would be admitted for a course of chemotherapy and follow the care outlined on that pathway. A second pathway for pain management might be started simultaneously.

3. Are the interventions on the pathway appropriate and acceptable to this patient's culture and desires? When the pathway was designed, it was not known if the patient using it would be a Native American, a Hmong, or an exchange student from China. These are all unique individuals with specific needs. Often nurses are hesitant to ask patients about their cultural wishes, not knowing the "right" words to use. While a comfort level will come with experience, be assured that patients are most often pleased and comforted by a nurse who makes an effort to meet those needs. One approach might be to say, "Do you have religious preferences or cultural practices that you would like to observe while you are in the hospital?" or "Could you tell me about your beliefs so that I can plan your nursing care to accommodate your beliefs as much as possible?"

4. What things need to be accomplished for the patient during this 8- or 12-hour shift, and which discipline is accountable for the intervention? The

IMPLEMENTATION

Listen, Understand, Act

*Sometimes the proper nursing intervention is simply to listen, under-
stand the patient's point of view, and explain the situation in a way that
can be understood by the patient.*

*I was called to our pediatric floor regarding a young Hmong fam-
ily whose small child needed emergency surgery for a burst appendix.
Knowing the Hmong culture as I did, I knew that it was going to be a
difficult conversation. Hmong people are reluctant to consent to surgery, have blood tests, or donate blood. They have a fear of cutting the
skin, thereby allowing potential evil spirits to invade the body, or, in the
case of the soul, allowing the body's good spirit to leave the body. The
parents were very concerned about the skin integrity and the potential
for evil spirits. I explained that I understood their desire not to have evil
spirits invade their child's body and that our hospital had a special place
where we did not allow evil spirits, "or what we call germs," to exist. This
place was the OR. I assured the parents that we took every precaution,
including having all of the staff wear masks, to avoid passing on any evil
spirit to their child. The parents finally consented to surgery.*

R. Peterson, RN, MSN

FIGURE 6-2.

nurse may note that the pathway indicates that the physical therapist will
ambulate a patient with a total hip replacement the first three times after
surgery. If the shift is half over and the therapist has not arrived, the nurse
may investigate and clarify the schedule. Similarly, if a physician consultation or diagnostic procedure was ordered for a patient and has not occurred,
the nurse may investigate and advocate for the patient. The coordination
function may save the patient unnecessary hospital days. This is not to say
that the nurse is responsible for "policing" other disciplines, but advocacy
and coordination are very much a part of the nursing role. These interventions are a part of every patient's nursing care whether or not a patient is on
a pathway.

SUMMARY

Implementation is the fifth step in the nursing process, and the focus is on the
nurse working with the patient and family to carry out the plan of care. Imple-

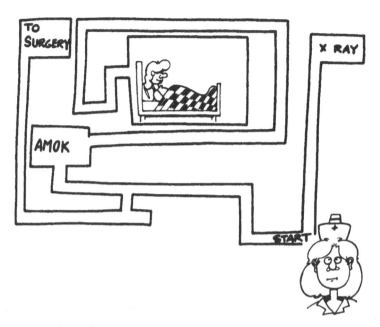

FIGURE 6-3.   Even the best-laid plans sometimes run amok.

mentation consists of validating the care plan (is it a safe, reasonable plan indicating high-quality nursing care?) and documenting and communicating it, but
the primary component is actually giving care to the patient. The nurse then documents this care and the patient's response to it in the chart. As the nurse gives
care, assessment of the patient continues. This is done not only to see how the
patient responds to the nursing interventions but also to provide increased information for revising the plan of care as patient status changes. The patient is an
active participant in care, working with the nurse to adapt interventions as they
are given and having the right to refuse or request interventions. The nurse is
flexible, open to suggestions and changing patient and family priorities, but
committed to helping them understand and accept nursing care to promote health
and reduce, eliminate, or prevent problems.

CRITICAL PATHWAY

Table 6-1 presents a critical pathway for a patient who is having total knee
replacement surgery. This table shows how the care might appear in the pathway
format. Table 6-2 is the patient version of a critical pathway that the nurse might
use as an educational tool for patients and families. Note that this version of the
pathway is written in lay language that would make it easy to understand without knowledge of medical vocabulary.

TABLE 6-1.

UW Health — TOTAL KNEE REPLACEMENT ORH 004

Admitting MD/Service _____
Primary Nurse _____ Associate Nurse _____
Allergies _____ Religion _____
Case Manager: _____
Admitting Diagnosis: _____
Operative Side: ☐ R ☐ L

Addressograph

Pt/family support systems; special considerations include: _____

History:

Significant Other (Name & Phone): _____

WORKING DIAGNOSIS DATE/TIME INTERVAL	/	D	Pre-op /	D E	Post-op /	D E	POD #1 /	N D E
UNIT SETTING	Learning Center/Ortho Clinic		FDS		B6/4		B6/4	
CONSULTS	Anesthesia						Physical Therapy	
LABS	CBC c̄ diff, Plt Chem survey, Lytes, PT, PTT, HIV, Sed Rate T&C ___ units		___ units Autologous blood available				Hct PT/PTT	
SPECIMENS (RN)	U/A - C/S				AP/Lat operative knee in PACU			
TESTS	CXR - ECG (if medically indicated or > 60 y.o.)							
ACTIVITY					ADLs c̄ assist Eating: Bathing: Activity: BR c̄ affected extremity↑ Knee in full extension & Ø pillow		ADLs c̄ assist Eating: Bathing: Activity: Affected extremity↑ Knee in full extension & Ø pillow Pivots to w/c c̄ leg ↑BID	

I = Independent
A = Assist (indicate amount needed)
D = Dependent

Indicate assistive devices

	VS ___	VS x 1 & PRN Void on call Pre-op checklist completed	VS q2°	VS q4°
T R E A T M E N T S *Call H.O. for:* T ___ P ___ R ___ BP ___ U.O. ___	Document : Functional Baseline Document CMS ___	Elastic stockings to unoperative leg to OR Document: Pre-op CMS baseline to affected extremity Health Care Profile in chart	CMS √q̄ ___ C&DB/IS q̄1°WA O_2 @ 2L √O_2 sat q̄ ___° titrate to keep O_2 sat ≥ ___% Elastic stocking SCDs (non-op leg) off 1° BID Ankle pump c̄ VS Retransfuse constavac within 6° post-op (by ___) per protocol Record drain output q̄8° St cath q̄6° if Ø VD I & O q̄8°	CMS √q̄4° C&DB/IS q̄1°WA O_2 @ ___ LPM √O_2 sat q̄ ___° titrate to keep O_2 sat ≥ ___% Pulse ox on RA Elastic stockings SCDs off 1° BID Ankle pump c̄ VS Knee immobilizer to affected leg when ↑ Retransfuse constavac within 6° post-op (by ___) per protocol Record drain output q̄8° Wean PCA St cath q̄6° if Ø VD I & O q̄8° until drain out & voiding spont. IV- D5.45 NaCl @ ___ cc/° ↓ as po ↑
D I E T	NPO	NPO	IV- D5.45 NS c̄ 20 KCl @ ___ cc/°	
			NPO Sips clear liquids if BS (+)	Advance diet as tolerated ___ (pre-admit diet)

Pt Name: ___ MR# ___

ORH 004 - 1

TABLE 6-1. (continued)

DISCHARGE PLANNING

Patient Health Profile:
Pt/family (Part I) completed ____
Nursing (Part II & III) completed ____
Residence: ____

Anticipated DC date: ____ Time: ____
Nursing Home/Other: ____
Phone: ____ Fax: ____
Transportation: ____
Phone: ____
LMD - FU: ____

Home services needed: RN ____ HHA ____
PT ____ OT ____ Other ____
Provider: ____
Phone: ____
Reason: ____

	D E	D	D E	D E	N D E
DATE					

NURSING / ACTIVITY & TEACHING

D E	D	D E	N D E
Assess: • level of pain • CMS √s to affected extremity	**Assess:** • complete systems x1 • CMS √s to affected extremity per standard & document baseline in narrative section of flowsheet	**Assess:** • complete systems q̄ 8° • level of pain q̄ 2° x 4 til then q̄ 4° • CMS √s to affected extremity q̄ 2° x 4	**Assess:** • complete systems q̄ 8° • level of pain q̄ 4° • CMS √s to affected extremity q̄ 4°

Teach Pt/Family: (date: ___)
• pain management/PCA
• autologous blood
• provide HFFY # 4864
• pre-op routines/restrictions
• LOS (length of stay)
• Advanced Directives
• a & during surgery:
  - post-op routine & equipment IS
  - DC & lifetime precautions
	Teach Pt/Family:
	• reinforce pre-op teaching
	• pt/family role in recovery:
	  - C & DB/IS
	  - activity
	  - DVT prophylaxis
	  - pain management
	  - PCA
		Teach Pt/Family:
		• post-op routines:
		  - DVT prophylaxis
		  - C&DB/IS
		• IV/fluid status
		• diet progression
		  - cath PRN
		• activity restrictions:
		  - bedrest c̄ operative leg ↑
		  - knee in full extension
		• pain management/PCA
		• review instructions & give controls when appropriate
		• medications: abx & anticoagulation
			Teach Pt/Family:
			• knee flexion & progression
			• activity to ↑ w/c BID
			• pain management, wean PCA to po
			• diet progression
			• review use of C & DB/IS
			• review isometric exercises

Other interventions: • discuss feelings of upcoming surgery		**Other interventions:** • listen to immediate concerns that pt/family express	**Other interventions:** • listen to pt/family concerns

172

OTHER DISCIPLINES ACTIVITY & TEACHING	**PT pre-op eval:** • assess baseline functional ability • exercises • TKA precautions • post-op PT schedule • modifications of home environment		**MD:** • communication c̄ family immediately post-op	**PT:** x2 @ bedside ___° knee flexion
ANTICIPATED VARIANCES		**Learning:** anxiety may impede learning **Support/Coping:** anxiety r/t surgery	**Cog:** sedated but recovering from anesthesia **Resp:** ↓ bases, clears c̄ C&DB/IS **GI:** Hypoactive bowel sounds **Funct:** BR needs assist c̄ ADLs & repositioning	**Learning:** level of fatigue may impede learning **Resp:** ↓ bases, clears c̄ C&DB/IS **GI:** hypoactive BS **Funct:** needs assist c̄ ADLs & max assist c̄ bed/chair transfers
OUTCOMES *(The pt/family will...)*	VS within MD parameters **Pts Pain Goal:**	VS within MD parameters **Pts Pain Goal:** Reports pain ≤ goal c̄ acceptable side effects	VS within MD parameters **Pts Pain Goal:** Reports pain ≤ goal c̄ acceptable side effects Drain ≤ 500cc q8° O₂ sat ≥ 92% Tolerates repositioning q2-4° c̄ assist	VS within MD parameters **Pts Pain Goal:** Reports pain ≤ goal c̄ acceptable side effects Tolerates cl liq s̄ N/V Tolerates chair 2x/d in AM & ↑ chair PM Drain c̄ ≤ 120cc/8° Flexes knee min 20° (if D.O.)
	Verbalize/Demonstrate: • LOS • understanding of pain management • how to prepare for knee surgery • what to expect during hospitalization • purpose & use of IS • a source of support while in hospital & @ home	**Verbalize/Demonstrate:** • progress anticipated • need for BR p̄ pre-op sedation • feelings/anxiety r/t surgery	**Verbalize/Demonstrate:** • correct use of PCA/ • Effective C&DB/IS • elastic stocking/ SCDs • Coping strategies consistent c̄ current health status	**Verbalize/Demonstrate:** • identifies 2 concerns re: rehab • correct use of IS, elastic stocking, SCDs • proper technique c̄ exercise program

Pt Name: _____ MR# _____

ORH 004 - 2   *Revised 05/06/98*

TABLE 6-1. (continued)

CODES:

√ = Within Parameter

* = Variance (does not meet parameter) AIR Note required for variances in the outcomes section

→ = Variance in patient condition unchanged

NR = Not Required

Date	Time	Initial & Signature	Date	Time	Initial & Signature

POD # 2 B6/4	N	D	E	POD # 3/ B6/4	N	D	E	POD # 4/ B6/4	N	D	E
OT (to begin POD#3)											
Hct				Hct							
PT/PTT				PT/PTT				PT/PTT			
ADLs c̄ assist				ADLs c̄ assist				ADLs c̄ assist			
Eating: 1				Eating: 1				Eating: 1			
Bathing: A mod				Bathing: A mod				Bathing: A min			
Activity:				Activity:				Activity:			
Pivots to w/c c̄ leg ↑				Pivots to w/c BID							
Amb ↑ c̄ walker & assist 2x/d				Amb ↑ c̄ walker to BR c̄ A 3x/d				Amb ↑ c̄ walker/ crutches c̄ stand by assist 3x/d min			

VS q̄ 4°	VS q̄ 4°	VS q̄ 8°
CMS √ q̄ 4°	CMS √ q̄ 4°	CMS √ q̄ 8°
C&DB/S q̄ 2-4° WA	C&DB/S q̄ 2-4° WA	C&DB/S PRN
Elastic stockings / SCD's / off 1° BID	Elastic stockings / SCD's / off 1° BID	Elastic stockings / SCD's / off 1° BID
Dry drsg Δ PRN (p̄ 1st Δ per MD order) / Record drain output q̄ 8° / d/c'd @ ___	Dry drsg Δ PRN	Dry drsg Δ PRN
Knee immobilizer to affected extremity when up	Knee immobilizer to affected extremity when up	
Dr. M: sling exercises QID / Dr. H: CPM speed - slowest / Extension 0 ___ / Flexion AM ___° / ADV to ___ PM ___°	Dr. M: sling exercises QID / Dr. H: CPM speed - slowest / Extension 0 ___ / Flexion AM ___° / ADV to ___ PM ___°	Dr. M: sling exercises QID / Dr. H: CPM speed - slowest
IV+heplwell		
Pre-admission diet	Pre-admission diet	Pre-admission diet

ORH 004 - 3   Pt Name: _____   MR# _____

TABLE 6-1. (continued)

☐ Plan DC prior to noon
Pt needs discussed at DC planning rounds on: _____

Referral called on: _____ by: _____

☐ DC supplies/equipment ordered
Referrals to: _____

Fax: _____
DME: _____
Vendor: _____
Phone: _____

	N	D	E		N	D	E		N	D	E
Assess:				**Assess:**				**Assess:**			
• level of pain q̄ 4°				• level of pain q 4°				• level of pain q 4°			
• CMS √s q̄ 4° to affected extremity				• CMS √s q̄ 4° to affected extremity				• CMS √s q 4° to affected extremity			
• GI q̄ 8 hrs				• GI → laxative if Ø stool							
• GU q̄ 8 hrs											
Teach Pt/Family:				**Teach Pt/Family:**				**Teach Pt/Family:**			
• sling exercises –Dr. M				• sn/sx of infection				• review HFFY			
• CPM instructions–Dr. H				• use of immobilizer				• restrictions upon DC			
• sn/sx of infections				• review sling exercise–Dr. M				• reinforce home exercise program (PT protocol)			
• constipation prevention				• review CPM–Dr. H				• review analgesics/meds for DC			
• po pain meds				• constipation prevention				• review TKA precautions per teaching guideline			
				• available DC resources				• when & who to call & what to report			
				• reinforce home exercise program (PT protocol)							
				• review TKA precautions per teaching guideline							
Other Interventions:				**Other Interventions:**				**Other Interventions:**			
• update DC plan				• discuss c̄ pt/family how surgery will affect home situation				• talk c̄ pt/family about coping strategies for life Δs @ home			
• discuss pt support system				• provide appropriate HFFY				• finalize DC plan			

176

PT:	PT:	Pharmacy: DC meds
° flexion ___ Ambulation ___ Equipment ___ Bed Mobility	° flexion ___ Ambulation ___ Equipment ___ Bed Mobility	PT: instruct family on activity ° flexion ___ Ambulation ___ Equipment ___ Bed Mobility
Funct: require assistive devices for amb (walker or crutches)	*Funct:* require assistive devices for amb (walker or crutches)	*Funct:* require assistive devices for amb (walker or crutches)
VS within MD parameters *Pts Pain Goal:* ___ Increasing knee flexion Ambulation in room c̄ mod assist Tolerates anxiety level app. to current health status	VS within MD parameters *Pts Pain Goal:* ___ Reports pain ≤ goal c̄ acceptable side effects Bowel movement since surgery Ambulates 50ft 2x/d, 1x/pm Increasing knee flexion	VS within MD parameters *Pts Pain Goal:* ___ Reports pain ≤ goal c̄ acceptable side effects Ø s/sx of infection Pt/family perceptions are consisent c̄ current health status @ D.C.
Verbalize/Demonstrate: • need for knee strengthening exercises • rationale for CPM • uses slings appropriately • identifies a source of emotional support	*Verbalize/Demonstrate:* • correct use of equipment • exercise protocols • Coping strategies effective for current health status	*Verbalize/Demonstrate:* • flexes knee min of 60° • knowledge of home exercise program • ambulates 100ft 2x/d, 1x/pm • Ds a way of dealing c̄ anticipated life Δs • DC plan & f/u care PT: DC criteria met

ORH 004-4   Pt Name: ___   MR# ___

TABLE 6-2.

UWHealth
University of Wisconsin Hospital and Clinics

Total Knee Replacement Pathway

* This pathway describes one course for a patient having Total Knee Replacement.
Your care and progress may vary to meet your needs. Discuss your progress with your nurse or case manager.

Today's Date	Clinic Visit	Day of Admission-Before Surgery	Day of Admission-After Surgery	1st Day after Surgery
Day				
Setting	Orthopedic Clinic & Learning Center	Orthopedics - B6/4	Orthopedics - B6/4	Orthopedics - B6/4
Activity	Your activity is not restricted unless you are told otherwise.	Remain on B6/4 until you go to surgery.	Bedrest with operated leg elevated and kept straight.	Begin Physical Therapy 2 times each day. Walk in room with assistance with walker or crutches. Use CPM or slings per your doctor.
Tests & Treatments	Blood tests Urinalysis Chest x-ray & Electrocardiogram (if you are 60 or older)	We will confirm any self donated blood. You will be asked to urinate before you leave for surgery. Your leg will again be scrubbed. Elastic stocking on your non-operative leg.	X-rays of your operated leg. Fluid intravenous (IV). Oxygen. Drain tube in operative knee. Knee immobilizer on operative leg. Elastic stocking and or compression device to your non-operative leg.	Blood tests. IV discontinued. Oxygen may be discontinued. Drain tube in operative knee. Knee immobilizer on operative leg. Elastic stockings and compression device to your non-operative leg.

Diet	Usual diet	No food or water	No food or water Possibly sips of liquid if your nurse determines you're ready for this.	Your usual diet
Teaching	Strengthening exercises & education on walker or crutches. You will be hospitalized 5 days, including day of surgery. How to prepare for surgery. How to manage pain after surgery. What to expect during your hospitalization. How to use the incentive spirometer. Support services in the hospital & at home.	Answer all of your questions. Support your family. Discuss your feeling about your upcoming surgery. Discuss your discharge plan.	Reinforce your post-surgery activities: - pain management - IV status - incentive spirometer - blood clot prevention - diet restrictions - activity restriction - medications We will listen to your questions & concerns	Knee flexion and progression Pain management Diet progression Review your incentive spirometer Talk about your concerns about rehabilitation

January 6, 1995 pw

Used with permission from UW Hospital and Clinics, Madison, Wisconsin.

UWHealth *University of Wisconsin Hospital and Clinics*

Total Knee Replacement Pathway - page 2

* This pathway describes one course for a patient having Total Knee Replacement.
Your care and progress may vary to meet your needs. Discuss your progress with your nurse or case manager.

Today's Date	2nd Day After Surgery	3rd Day After Surgery	4th Day After Surgery		
Day					
Setting	Orthopedics - B6/4	Orthopedics - B6/4	Orthopedics - B6/4, then home		
Activity	Physical Therapy 2 times. Walk in room with assistance with walker or crutches. Use CPM or slings per your doctor.	Physical Therapy 2 times. Walk 50 feet 3 times. Use walker or crutches properly. Bend knee further.	Physical Therapy - can walk safely 100 feet with walker or crutches and understand home exercise program. Bend knee at least 60°.		
Tests & Treatments	Blood tests. Drain tube discontinued. Knee immobilizer on operative leg. Elastic stockings and compression device to your non-operative leg.	Blood tests. Knee immobilizer on operative leg. Elastic stockings and compression device to your non-operative leg.	Blood tests. Knee immobilizer on operative leg. Elastic stockings to be worn at home every day until most of the swelling has resolved.		

180

Diet	Your usual diet	Your usual diet	Your usual diet
Teaching	Continuous Passive Motion (CPM) or sling instruction based on your doctor's orders. Constipation prevention. Update your discharge plan. Continue with activity instructions.	Signs and symptoms of infection. How to use your immobilizer. Review the total knee replacement precaution. Identify appropriate resources at home. Reinforce your home exercise program.	Review "Health Facts For You". Review activities and medications. Identify who and when to call; what to report. Identify ways of dealing with life changes. Confirm your discharge plan.

181

Evaluation

Evaluation occurs continuously while care is being given, shift by shift, as nurses evaluate progress toward intermediate outcomes and summatively at discharge from the health care facility with the evaluation of discharge outcomes. There are four distinct activities in the evaluation phase of the nursing process.

	Documenting	Evaluating	Evaluating	Reviewing
Evaluating =	Responses to Interventions	+ Effectiveness of Interventions	+ Outcome Achievement	+ Nursing Care Plan

DOCUMENTING RESPONSES TO INTERVENTIONS

While giving care to the patient, the nurse continually evaluates the patient's response to the interventions. The patient may be responding in the way the nurse expected—the way most patients respond. In this situation the nursing treatment or action produced the expected result, and the nurse will describe this response in the patient's chart or on whatever form of documentation the health care facility is using: "Patient tolerated standing at bedside and walking to bathroom with only minor dizziness on first ambulation postoperatively."

Perhaps the patient responded in an unexpected way, either positively or negatively. The nurse documents this response too but usually has to adapt the subsequent interventions planned because of this unexpected response. The alteration in subsequent interventions is then documented along with the patient's response: "Patient became very dizzy and slightly nauseated when standing at bedside while attempting first ambulation postop. Patient returned to bed. Instructed not to attempt getting out of bed without assistance." Now the nurse has to select new nursing interventions on the spot, based on these patient reactions to the attempted ambulation. The nurse assesses the vital signs, gives the patient a cool washcloth for the face, and reassures the patient that this response is not unusual and that the next attempt will go better. The nurse shares the modified plan to delay ambulating again until the patient has had a chance to take in some food and fluids over the next few hours. For safety, the nurse emphasizes that the patient should not attempt to get out of bed without a nurse to help. This is an example of the kind of ongoing evaluation and adaptation of the planned interventions that goes on continually while a nurse is giving care. All aspects of this process are documented: the action(s), the patient response(s) and the adaptations made in the interventions, and later the patient response(s) after the implementation of the adapted interventions.

EVALUATING THE EFFECTIVENESS OF INTERVENTIONS

A nurse using the nursing process is always aware of the intermediate and discharge outcomes selected as goals for patient behaviors after nursing interventions. These outcomes are the criteria on which evaluation is based. Interventions are evaluated in terms of their usefulness in assisting the patient to move toward these outcomes. Nursing interventions are based on scientific principles and nursing knowledge. They are supposed to produce a specific result when used with most patients. If the nursing interventions produce the expected result in patient behavior, they are effective and will advance the patient toward the desired outcome. If the interventions produce an unexpected result or are not possible to implement at the expected time because of variations in a patient's response or speed of recovery, the interventions need to be examined to try to improve their effectiveness. Questions the nurse can ask as interventions are evaluated include the following:

1. Was there a language barrier or cultural orientation of the nurse, the patient, or the family that reduced the effectiveness of the intervention? What can be done to remedy this?
2. Do I need more skill or practice to make this intervention more effective?
3. Did I consider approaching the problem from many different angles, or did I use only one intervention (for example, giving an analgesic when

requested by the patient versus exploration of the pain to try to eliminate precipitating factors combined with other pain management strategies in addition to medication)?

4. Would my interventions be more effective if the family or significant others were more involved? Less involved?
5. Did I share the plan with the patient to promote understanding and participation?
6. Do I need to seek out the expertise of another nurse to suggest interventions, adaptations of interventions, or resequencing of interventions that would be more effective?
7. Did the patient's condition change, making the type and timing of the interventions less appropriate and therefore less effective?

EVALUATION OF OUTCOME ACHIEVEMENT

The purpose of this part of the evaluation is to determine whether the patient has achieved the outcomes selected during the outcome identification phase of the nursing process. The outcomes are evaluated at the time or date specified in the plan. While giving care, the nurse continuously collects new data about the patient. Some of this information will be used for evaluation of outcome achievement. When evaluating outcome achievement, the nurse returns to the outcome statement in the care plan. What was the specific patient behavior stated in the desired outcome? Was the patient able to perform the behavior by the time allowed in the outcome statement? Was the patient able to perform the behavior as well as described in the criteria part of the outcome statement? The answers to these questions form the basis for an evaluation of outcome achievement.

The only thing that is evaluated is the patient's ability to demonstrate the behavior described in the outcome statement. Nursing actions are not evaluated at this point and are not part of the evaluation statement. Effectiveness of the nursing actions and teaching plans will be examined separately. The nurse may have given the world's fastest bedbath, but that is not important for evaluating outcome achievement. If the intermediate outcome was to have the patient relax and sleep for several hours, the nurse evaluates the resulting patient behavior. Did the patient sleep for several hours? The skill with which a nurse performs various procedures is important and will affect outcome achievement. However, when an evaluative statement is written, it is the patient's behavior or condition that is assessed. *The result of nursing care in the form of changed patient behavior or condition is the focus of outcome-based, criterion-referenced evaluation.*

Patient Participation and Evaluation

Evaluation of outcome achievement is done with the patient and family whenever possible. It also may be done with other health care providers as appropri-

ate. It is not just the nurse's assessment of the patient's ability to achieve an outcome that is important. The patient's perception is also important since the problem identified in the nursing diagnosis is the patient's problem, not the nurse's. The patient who evaluates personal outcome achievement is a partner with the nurse and receives feedback on progress toward eliminating or reducing the original problem identified in the nursing diagnosis. When a patient successfully achieves an outcome mutually set with the nurse, that patient receives positive reinforcement to continue efforts toward a higher level of functioning.

Writing an Evaluative Statement

There are two parts to an evaluative statement: a decision on how well the outcome was achieved, and the patient data or behavior that support that decision. The nurse has three alternatives when deciding how well an outcome was met: (1) met, (2) partially met, and (3) not met.

If the patient was able to demonstrate the behavior by the specific time or date in the outcome statement, the outcome was met. If the patient was able to demonstrate the behavior but not as well as the nurse had specified in the outcome statement, the outcome was partially met. If the patient was unable or unwilling to perform the behavior at all, the outcome was not met.

Outcome Evaluation Statement	=	Outcome Met Outcome Partially Met Outcome Not Met	+	Actual Patient Behavior as Evidence

In the second part of the evaluation statement, the nurse includes a description of the patient's actual behavior as the individual tries to demonstrate the behavior identified in the outcome. For example, if the behavior identified in the outcome was for the patient to report some degree of pain relief, the nurse talks with the patient regarding severity of pain following the nursing interventions to help relieve it. The patient's response about the severity of current pain makes up the second part of the outcome evaluative statement. Other examples might be the following:

1. Nursing Diagnosis: Activity intolerance related to prolonged bed rest.
   Outcome Statement: Patient will walk length of hall and back by 2/7.
   Outcome Evaluation (done on 2/7 or earlier):
   Outcome achieved; patient walked length of hall and back.
   Outcome partially achieved; patient walked length of hall but too tired to walk back.
   Outcome not achieved; patient refused to walk because of nausea.
   Outcome not achieved; patient unable to bear his own weight.
2. Nursing Diagnosis: Impaired tissue integrity related to pressure and poor circulation.

Outcome Statement: 2/7: Decubitus ulcer (bed sore) will be healed in 1 month.

Outcome Evaluation (done on 3/7 or earlier):

Outcome met; decubitus ulcer healed.

Outcome partially met; decubitus ulcer still present but is 1/2 the size.

Outcome not met; decubitus ulcer broken open and draining.

3. Nursing Diagnosis: Noncompliance with assigned reading in *Understanding the Nursing Process* related to belief that content is "boring."

Outcome Statement: After finishing Chapter 7, the student will state that this nursing process book is the most interesting book ever read.

Outcome Evaluation (done when the student finishes Chapter 7):

Outcome met; student stated this book was the most interesting book ever read and asked for an "A" in the course.

Outcome partially met; student said this book was about as interesting as any other course books and asked for a "C" in the course.

Outcome not met; student lost book and asked for a class withdrawal slip.

When evaluating outcome achievement, the nurse is responsible for documenting both parts of the outcome statement. The nurse doing the evaluation with the patient includes the date the evaluation was done, the degree to which the outcome was achieved, subjective and objective data related to the patient's

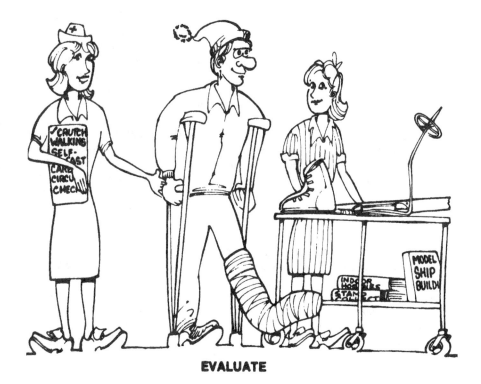

EVALUATE

FIGURE 7-1.   Discharge outcome achieved. Congratulations!

TABLE 7-1   EVALUATION OF OUTCOMES

Nursing Diagnoses	Outcomes	Outcome Evaluation
1. Knowledge deficit of diabetic management related to new diagnosis	1. Maintains control of blood glucose levels from 80–180 m/dl (long-term outcome) a. accurately checks blood glucose level qid before discharge (discharge outcome)	a. outcome met; correctly performed self blood glucose checks × 4 *L. Atkinson R.N.*
	b. lists signs and symptoms of hyperglycemia and hypoglycemia by 11/12 (intermediate outcome)	b. outcome partially met; lists S&S for hypoglycemia, confused on hyperglycemia *L. Atkinson R.N.*
	c. states actions to take for hyper/hypoglycemia by 11/12 (intermediate outcome)	c. outcome met; stated corrective actions for hyper/hypoglycemia *L. Atkinson R.N.*
	d. correctly administers own insulin by discharge (discharge outcome)	d. outcome met; correctly gave self mixed dose of NPH and regular insulin × 2 days *L. Atkinson R.N.*
	e. correctly explains how to adjust diet and insulin with short-term illness by 11/13 (intermediate outcome)	e. outcome not met; states never sick and does not think adjustment necessary *L. Atkinson R.N.*
2. Fear related to development of diabetes and complications that may develop	2. States decreased fear and confidence in ability to reduce risks of complications by 11/14 (long-term outcome)	2. Outcome met. States, "It will be a constant worry, but I am not as terrified as I was. Lots of people do fine managing their diabetes." *L. Atkinson R.N. 12/14/00*
3. Body image disturbance related to diagnosis of Type 1 diabetes as evidenced by anger over need to take insulin and change life-style	3. Verbalizations of acceptance of diab. and willingness to make changes by 12/14 (long-term outcome)	3. Outcome not met; patient states anger about dx and states it's not fair. "I just hate taking shots; it makes me feel like a drug addict." *L. Atkinson R.N. 12/14/00*

behavior compared to the behavior identified in the outcome, and the nurse's signature. This information is all recorded on the chart or care plan. See Table 7-1.

REVIEW OF THE NURSING CARE PLAN

After evaluation of outcome achievement, the nurse repeats the activities in the nursing process by reviewing the plan of care. This is done whether the outcome was achieved or not. Review of the nursing care plan keeps the plan current and responsive to the patient's changing needs. The process of nursing is not just sequential, consisting of steps 1 through 6 and then you are done. The process of nursing is cyclical in nature, with the steps of assessment, diagnosis, outcome identification, planning, implementation, and evaluation viewed as a circle with one step leading to another. The nursing care a person receives reflects the changing health status of the patient, medical treatment changes, environmental changes, and the changing needs of the patient and family.

Review of the Nursing Care Plan	=	Reassessment	+	Review of Nursing Diagnoses	+	Review of Outcomes and Replanning	+	Review of Implementation

Review of the care plan using the nursing process consists of activities already described in the previous chapters: reassessment, review of diagnoses, review of outcomes, replanning, and review of implementation. This process of review results in an updated plan for nursing care, which is then implemented and evaluated, leading again to review as part of evaluation.

Reassessment

The process of reassessment results in an updated information base on the patient. The nurse continually assesses the patient during all interactions. This accumulation of new data will now supplement the original data base from which the care plan was developed. After evaluation of intermediate outcome achievement, the nurse looks at the data, diagnoses, desired outcomes, and interventions again. In reassessment, the nurse

1. Examines original data (related to the problem and intermediate outcome just evaluated) to decide whether they still accurately represent the patient's status.
2. Examines new data gathered during interventions with the patient to clarify the original problem, its etiology, and related signs and symptoms and to serve as a data base for new nursing diagnoses.

Review of Nursing Diagnoses

The end product of reviewing the nursing diagnoses is a care plan containing only those diagnoses that are current or risk problems for the patient. This may result in the same diagnoses continuing as part of the plan, new diagnoses being added, and resolved diagnoses being eliminated. During the process of reviewing diagnoses, the nurse

1. Analyzes new data to determine whether a new problem exists and makes a new nursing diagnosis as needed. This addition is then documented in the care plan.
2. Analyzes original and new data, including data from outcome evaluation, to determine whether the original diagnoses are still accurate, current problems requiring nursing care. If they are still accurate and current, these diagnoses remain on the care plan as originally written.
3. Clarifies diagnostic statements to reflect any changes or additions in etiology or signs and symptoms discovered during ongoing assessment with the patient. These changes are then added to the original diagnostic statement in the chart.
4. Analyzes original and new data and data from outcome evaluation to determine whether the problem has been resolved and no longer requires nursing care. "Diagnosis resolved" is then documented and dated on the chart, and nurses no longer perform the interventions associated with that diagnosis.

If the outcome was not achieved, reassessment and review of the diagnoses may help point out the reasons for this, such as inaccurate or incomplete data, inaccurate analysis of the data resulting in an invalid nursing diagnosis, and the development of new problems that interfered with the original plan. If the outcome was met and the problem was resolved, the nurse considers the need for preventive nursing care if the patient is still at risk.

A student in nursing discovers the problem when review of the care plan is not complete . . .

I was teaching with a group of third-quarter nursing students on an orthopedic clinical area. We had spent a lot of classroom and clinical time developing nursing care plans, but in the actual clinical setting the students found standard care plans being used. Nurses would diagnose a problem area based on patient assessment and then use the NANDA-approved diagnoses with suggested goals and interventions all typed out. The nurse was to individualize this care plan based on knowledge of the patient and the medical treatment plan and put it in the chart. Well, the students were thrilled. This was a lot better than creating a care plan

from scratch. A few words and marks on a preprinted form and they were done. One student in particular was irritated with the nursing faculty for making the students do all this work of care planning when in reality the nurses in the hospital were using care plan forms developed by experienced nurses from the health care facility. The Kardex contained only a list of partially written diagnoses such as "Pain" or "Impaired Physical Mobility." I expressed my concern that care plan review could easily be neglected by such a process because many nurses do not use the chart as a guide to nursing care but continue to use the Kardex, which no longer contains the plan of care. My fears were dismissed as unrealistic because on the flow sheet in the patient's chart each shift documented, by initialing, that the care plan had been reviewed. About an hour later, that student called me over and said she had a real problem. The patient she had been caring for all shift was 4-days postop with an amputation. The student had found the plan of care and knew she had to read it because I would be around asking if it was updated. The diagnosis of "Pain related to poor circulation and skin breakdown areas on left lower leg" was still in the chart as originally individualized by the admitting nurse over a week ago. That lower leg had been amputated 4 days ago. "How could this happen?" she asked. I just smiled. The students had a great postconference discussion on charting, care planning, legal documentation, and ethics.

Review of Outcomes and Replanning

The result of this activity will be a plan of care ready for implementation based on current problems, with outcomes and interventions adjusted to best reflect the patient's abilities and preferences. Ineffective interventions can be eliminated, effective ones emphasized, and new approaches included to facilitate movement toward the achievement of discharge outcomes. During this step, the nurse

1. Reexamines priorities among the diagnoses and determines whether they are still appropriate. Priorities are reordered as needed based on new data, new diagnoses, medical management, and expected date for discharge, transfer, surgery, and so on.
2. Examines previous outcomes and determines whether they are still appropriate or if the patient's status has changed, making the outcomes unrealistic. The behavior, time frame, criteria, and condition can all be altered to make the intermediate outcomes and discharge outcomes more appropriate and achievable while still moving toward problem resolution.
3. Identifies new outcomes for new diagnoses and selects interventions. These then are documented in the chart.

4. Examines nursing interventions selected in the original plan and determines whether they should continue unchanged or whether a different approach would be more effective. Any changes, additions, or deletions are then documented in the chart as part of the updated care plan.

Without reassessment by a nurse, the client's recovery may have been at risk . . .

I hate to float to another area when our floor isn't busy. But float me they did. I usually worked on the burn unit and really felt competent working with the patients, but they floated me to an oncology/chemotherapy unit. Different treatments, different problems, different things to assess, lots of drugs to look up. One of my patients was a man admitted to the hospital for workup of an unidentified blood disorder that had been causing him trouble for 15 years. The focus of care was on his hematologic problem, pain management, and possible narcotic addiction. On the Kardex it was noted that he had a partial-thickness burn on the palm of his hand that had been treated in the emergency room. The last date on the treatment order for the burn was a week ago. I knew what a burn of that degree should look like if it was healing properly, but his hand didn't look the way it should. I assessed the hand and reviewed the ordered treatment based on my own knowledge of burn healing, complications, and available treatments. I discussed my concerns with the head nurse, who admitted being unfamiliar with burn therapy and complications. She notified the responsible physician, who then asked for a consultation from one of the physicians on the burn unit. The doctor came down and reassessed the burn and the treatment and told me it was a good thing I had questioned the healing and treatment. He said I had probably saved the patient from an infection and possible sepsis by my assessment and action. I guess some days nurses are meant to float.

The following example illustrates review of the plan of care. The readers should understand that these steps are not written out as such in the plan as are diagnoses, outcomes, and interventions; the plan of care is continually updated, using whatever form of documentation the health care setting has implemented. Therefore, the nurse will not find the headings of "reassessment," "review of diagnoses," "review of plan," and "review of implementation" as part of the care plan. These steps indicate the *process* the nurse goes through to reach the *product* of an effective, current plan of care.

Nursing Diagnoses	Outcome	Interventions	Outcome Evaluation
At risk for impaired tissue integrity r/t cast on left leg 6/4/00	Tissue to remain intact, with normal sensation, while hospitalized in cast	1. Assess CMS qh × 24 then q4h 2. Elevate leg in good alignment × 24h 3. Turn and reposition q2h until cast dry 4. Pad friction areas at knee and toes	Date: 6/6/00 Outcome met; tissue intact at discharge

Developed by: *L. Atkinson R.N. 6/4/00*

Signature of nurse evaluating: *L. Atkinson R.N. 6/6/00*

New Data	New Updated Outcome	New Interventions
1. 6/6 discharge to home in cast. 2. Skin intact at discharge. (Original Dx still appropriate)	Tissue to remain intact, with normal sensation while casted	1. Assess knowledge of S&S of inadeq circ., pressure, friction 2. Teach home care of cast 3. Enc. elevation when sitting at home/work

Developed by: *L. Atkinson R.N. 6/6/00*

Review of Implementation

During review of implementation, the nurse examines what actually happened with the patient and family during nursing care. Factors such as the environment, the nurse's skills and knowledge, and the patient's and family's responses are considered. This is where the nurse evaluates personal behavior in relation to giving care. Does the nurse require further skills or information to be more effective? Did the nurse's personal feelings or cultural bias affect the quality of care delivered? Were the interventions realistic in terms of time and resources? Were

the interventions carried out by other nursing or health care personnel? If not, why not? Were the interventions too vague or misinterpreted? Review of what occurred during implementation of the original nursing plan of care may point out problems that can be corrected as the plan is updated. This is especially important when the intermediate outcome or discharge outcome was not achieved. Evaluation helps the nurse develop the skills of writing realistic and effective care plans for dealing with a patient's problems.

CRITICAL THINKING FOR EVALUATION

During this phase of the nursing process the nurse uses criterion-based evaluation. The behavior identified in the outcome statement is the criterion for judging the resulting patient behavior. This is a critical-thinking skill. A critical thinker seeks objective and subjective patient data to judge the effectiveness of the original assessments, diagnosis, outcome, plan, and implementation. Depending on the findings from this reflective process, the nurse may have to correct her or his thinking and reexamine the whole plan. This is the truth-seeking step where the nurse and patient compare the actual outcome to the planned outcome.

The whole patient is reassessed after implementation. Are there new cues from the patient that lead you to suspect a new problem? What was the impact of the plan on the patient's health status? For example, the nurse and patient may have met their pain management outcome of a rating of 4 or less on a pain scale of 1–10, but the level of consciousness decreased to the point where the patient could not stay awake and felt "too drugged." A critically thinking nurse will reflect on the plan with a new dual purpose in mind: pain control with less sedation. Knowledge, experience, new information, and sound reasoning skills will help the nurse amend the plan to better fit the patient's needs, and the nurse will try again.

All the parts of the nursing process are viewed as interrelated by a critically thinking nurse, and changes in one area are anticipated to affect all other areas. They will be reexamined for appropriateness. The nurse is constantly thinking, "So what?" and "Now what?" Outcomes that were not met may require additional documentation. This requires time, energy, honesty, and integrity. The nurse often is expected to develop and document a new plan that will be more likely to succeed, and this process requires creativity and possibly additional resources or information. A nurse who is a critical thinker takes responsibility for all this, confident that a new and better plan can be developed.

Prompts for Critical Thinking during Evaluation

- Were your evaluations of outcome achievement accurate? What was your evidence?

- Are there any new problems? Do you need more data to confirm this?
- Did the interventions help the patient achieve the desired outcomes? Do the patient and family agree? Do other health care providers agree?
- What is the clinical significance of the resulting patient status? Is the patient better?
- Will the patient's resulting status affect the plan? How?
- Why did the plan work so well? Can you replicate it?
- Why did the plan not succeed in achieving the outcome? Can you correct that and prevent it from happening again?
- How could things have been done differently to achieve even better out-comes?
- Were there assumptions, biases, or points of view that you missed? What effect did that have on outcome achievement and the entire plan?
- What are you going to do differently next time? Why?
- "So what? Now what?"

CULTURALLY COMPETENT NURSING CARE DURING EVALUATION

When evaluating the patient's progress toward a health care outcome, the nurse can examine several aspects. If the nurse was successful in helping the patient achieve the outcome in the plan of care, examine why. Why did it go so well this time? Did cultural information and considerations contribute to success? Always be alert to finding a more effective, timely way of doing something with similar patients who have similar problems and try to replicate your success.

If the patient was unable to achieve the outcome in a timely manner, was the outcome realistic for this patient, from this culture, with this time orientation, and with these cultural beliefs about health, disease, and treatments? Was there congruence between the Western medicine treatment plan and the patient's cultural expectations, values, and beliefs? Could the plan have been developed to include more cultural practices that this patient and family believe in and find comforting?

If the patient did not seem pleased with the care and treatments received regardless of whether outcomes were achieved, explore the accuracy of your interpretation with the patient: "You do not seem pleased about your progress. Is there something wrong or something that is bothering you?" "Your family seems upset. Are they concerned about the treatment you are getting here?" "What would make you feel more comfortable with your care and how your problems are being treated?"

If you found yourself getting irritated during care delivery, try to identify why. Did it take more time? Did the family or patient require more explanations? Did it take more effort and thinking on your part? Was it just plain crowded?

Then try to understand the special meaning any care adaptations had for this patient and family. These could be the most important of all to them when they look back on the quality of the care received.

As part of evaluation, the nurse may identify a personal knowledge and skill deficit related to working with patients from a particular culture. Seek out the information and skills you need through the Internet, cultural workshops, professional journals, and people from the culture. Ask your patients for suggestions: "I work with many patients and their families from Somalia, and sometimes I think they are very pleased with their care but other times I think we could do better. Do you or your family have any suggestions for us? Anything that you think would have been helpful to your recovery?"

Try, Try Again

In evaluating a patient's outcomes, there may be times when the plan of care has failed. A plan can fail for many reasons. Not taking a patient's culture into account can be one of those reasons. When I was a young nurse on an oncology floor, I was caring for a Taiwanese woman with advanced liver cancer. She was in a great amount of pain, which concerned me. The first morning, in the middle of her bath, I noticed she was wearing what I learned were Chinese pain patches all over her abdomen. Not believing that those patches could really help her, I spent several days trying to persuade her to use morphine. She refused, believing that the patches would work. During the next few days her pain increased, but she continued to refuse the morphine. I spoke with her husband about using pain medication because I did not want her to die in pain. He explained the importance of the patches both within their religious context and from a cultural standpoint. He asked me if I would please believe in the patches, if not for me, at least for his wife's sake. I agreed, but with my nursing background it was difficult. Within a day or so she died. I spent a long time wondering if the outcome would have been different if she had tried the morphine. It wasn't until years later that I began to understand where my plan had gone wrong. I had discounted my patient's values, beliefs, and convictions. I could have thought more creatively and combined my knowledge of pain management with her beliefs. Could the morphine analgesic patches have met her needs? I never even considered it.

R. Peterson, RN, MSN

Prompts for Culturally Competent Nursing Care during Evaluation

- Was there a language barrier that could have been handled more effectively?
- Did the original assessment include enough cultural content to help the nurse be sensitive to cultural needs when developing the plan of care?
- Did the diagnoses consider cultural factors in problem definition or contributing etiology?
- Did the patient view the diagnoses as problems from his or her cultural perspective?
- Did outcomes consider this individual's cultural expectations for recovery?
- Did the plan include cultural components to make the patient feel comfortable, secure, and respected?
- Was care delivered in a nondiscriminatory, nonjudgmental manner?

EVALUATION: THE MANAGED CARE ENVIRONMENT

Evaluation of clinical outcomes on critical pathways occurs on two levels: the level of the individual patient and the aggregate or group level. When a nurse is caring for an individual patient, the pathway specifies a time for the evaluation of a clinical outcome. For example, the patient should be able to walk 50 feet the first day postop. The patient, Mrs. Jones, may be extremely nauseated and vomiting after a sleepless night. The nurse notes this change from the expected outcome on the critical pathway. This change is called an individual variance. Each variance is unexpected and requires that the nurse make a progress note. While the format of the notes varies in different institutions, each note must incorporate the nurse's assessment of the patient, a statement of a plan to modify the patient's condition, and a reassessment after the plan has been implemented. This modification of the pathway is designed to individualize a plan of care when the patient has outcomes and/or time frames different from those on the pathway. The goal of the modified plan would be to get the patient back "on track," back to the plan of care on the critical pathway. One of the advantages of using critical pathways is that variances from clinical outcomes are quickly identified by the nurse and the plan of care then is modified.

Not all variances from the critical pathway are bad. Some patients may progress at a much faster rate and deviate from the pathway in a positive direction. It is equally important to note these changes from the pathway. Was there something the patient or the nurse did that could be used to help other patients? What can we learn from these patients?

At the group or aggregate level nurses are interested in variances from expected outcomes. Variance data often are collected from patient records as part of quality improvement projects. Each variance is noted and classified according to one of three categories:

1. Systems problem: The patient was not scheduled for a magnetic resonance image (MRI) because the test is not done on the weekend unless it is an emergency.
2. Provider problem: Dr. Jones had a full surgery schedule, and the patient had to wait 48 hours.
3. Patient problem: Mrs. Smith was 95 years old, frail, and unable to tolerate movement after surgery.

As the data from variance notes are collected and analyzed, quality improvement teams may identify projects that would improve patient care. For example, what would it take to have MRI routinely available on weekends? How much would it cost? How many unnecessary patient days were there because the test was not available? One quality improvement project that is frequently reported in the literature is the delay in getting intravenous (IV) antibiotics started for pneumonia patients admitted from the emergency department (ED). This is a systems issue that involves several disciplines and various hospital departments. If the desired outcome is that antibiotics be started within 4 hours of an ED admission and variance notes indicate that this routinely takes 6 to 8 hours, a quality improvement team might begin to investigate the process and plan needed changes. This improvement in patient care is based on grouped data that nurses have documented in the chart. Many hospitals routinely share these data with staff nurses, who are in an excellent position to use the information to improve patient care.

SUMMARY

Evaluation involves four activities. Documenting patient responses to interventions and evaluating the effectiveness of those interventions are the first two activities. Another part of evaluation involves evaluation of outcome achievement. To do this, the nurse returns to the outcome to review the behavior identified that would indicate a lessening or elimination of an actual patient problem. Using the new data collected during implementation of the care plan, the nurse, patient, and family whenever possible evaluate the patient's ability to demonstrate the outcome behavior. A range of outcomes can be expected, from com-

plete ability to demonstrate the behavior as stated to complete inability or unwillingness to demonstrate the behavior. This evaluation is documented in the chart with a description of the patient's outcome behavior as evidence of the degree of achievement.

The last part of evaluation is to review the entire plan of care. This involves updating the data base, deciding if original diagnoses are still accurate, adding new diagnoses or identifying original ones as resolved, revising the outcomes and interventions on the basis of more complete information on the patient and the effectiveness of the original plan, and finally implementing the updated plan. This is again followed by evaluation and care plan review to reflect the dynamic state of the patient (see Figure 7-2).

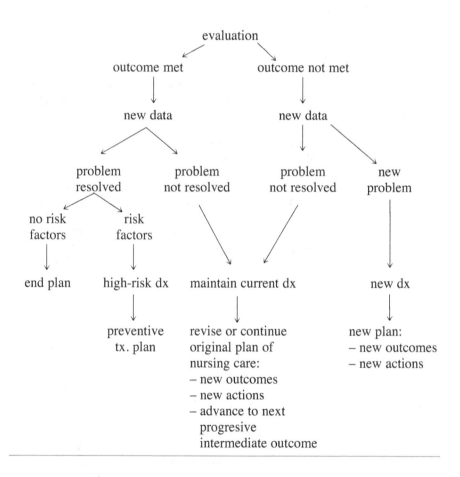

FIGURE 7-2. Evaluation flow chart.

CASE STUDY: EVALUATION

The case study of Mrs. Wiley is continued to illustrate the evaluation of a plan of care.

EVALUATION #1
PREOPERATIVE ORTHOPEDIC SURGERY CLINIC

Mrs. Wiley: Evaluation of the plan of care is done by the nurse in the orthopedic clinic before surgery.

Nursing Diagnoses	Clinical Outcomes	Interventions	Evaluation
Knowledge deficit: strengthening exercises, crutch walking, pain management after surgery, use of incentive spirometer, preoperative preparation for surgery	Verbalize/-demonstrate: strengthening exercises, anticipated length of stay (LOS), what to expect during hospitalization, understanding of pain management and pain rating scale, use of incentive spirometer, crutch walking.	Teach patient and family: 1. Pain management after surgery (PCA). 2. Preoperative routines/instructions. 3. Offer advance directives. 4. Equipment: continuous passive motion machine (CPM). 5. Refer to home health nursing for home assessment. 6. Refer to physical therapy to teach crutch walking.	Outcome partially met. Patient and family participated in teaching program and state understanding of surgery, pain management (PCA), LOS, spirometer, CPM. Mrs. Wiley unsteady on crutches after following PT instructions. States understanding of general postop course for total knee replacement surgery and activity restrictions. Home health nursing assessment complete. *M. Knedle, RN 10/17/00*
Husband: risk for injury related to absence of care provider	Husband will remain injury-free during absence and recovery of primary caregiver (Mrs. Wiley).	1. Discuss/clarify need with patient and husband. 2. Document and communicate needs to home health nurse.	Unable to evaluate at this time. Plan for family member to stay in home for 2 weeks, assisted by home health care agency. *M. Knedle, RN 10/17/00*

Nursing Diagnoses	Clinical Outcomes	Interventions	Evaluation
Chronic pain related to degeneration of knee joint	Patient will state that pain is controlled at 4 or less on activity or less than 2 at rest until time of surgery.	1. Assess what Mrs. Wiley is taking, how frequently, and level of relief. 2. Communicate pain relief need to physician. 3. Instruct patient about new med. 4. Teach noninvasive pain control: cold, distraction, relaxation tapes.	Outcome met. States pain has been 4 or less most of the time and 2 at rest. *M. Knedle, RN 10/17/00*

EVALUATION #2
FIRST DAY SURGERY CENTER: 7 A.M.

Patients are admitted to the first day surgery center the morning of surgery for their scheduled procedures and are transferred to the inpatient unit after surgery.

Mrs. Wiley: Evaluation of the plan of care is done by the nurse at the time Mrs. Wiley leaves the preoperative area on the day of surgery.

Nursing Diagnoses	Clinical Outcomes	Interventions	Evaluation
Fear of reduced mobility related to outcome of surgery	Patient will report reduced fear levels before leaving preop prep area.	1. Encourage patient to verbalize clarify/ fears. 2. Have family member/nurse remain with patient until patient goes to OR. 3. Share experience of typical patient with this surgery and outcomes of less pain and more mobility. 4. Offer comfort measures: warm blanket, pillows.	Outcome met. "It helped to talk about it and know that other people have done well." "Having less pain and more movement would really be wonderful." *J. E. Murray, RN 10/29/00*

Nursing Diagnoses	Clinical Outcomes	Interventions	Evaluation
Risk for injury (Mrs. Wiley) related to lack of experience with crutch walking	Patient will be injury-free during hospitalization and home recovery.	1. Communicate to nurse on postop unit in writing and on care plan. 2. Teach crutch walking on flat surface and on stairs before discharge.	Unable to eval. at this time. *J. E. Murray, RN 10/29/00*
Anxiety (patient and family members) related to surgical experience	Patient and family will demonstrate reduced anxiety within 6 hours.	1. Orient family members to waiting area, cafeteria. 2. Give written phone number of post-operative unit, assigned post-operative room and phone number. 3. Tell them how, where, and when they will obtain information. 4. Offer beverages and/or directions to cafeteria.	Unable to eval. at this time. *J. E. Murray, RN 10/29/00*

EVALUATION #3
POSTOPERATIVE ORTHOPEDIC PATIENT CARE UNIT

Mrs. Wiley: Evaluation of the plan of care is done by the nurse on postoperative orthopedic surgery unit.

Nursing Diagnoses	Clinical Outcomes	Interventions	Evaluation
Acute pain related to joint replacement surgery, movement, and physical therapy	Pain will remain at 3 or less throughout hospitalization.	1. Assess pain at least every 2 hours. 2. Reinforce teaching on PCA pump. 3. Record pain intensity, intervention, response.	Outcome partially met. When pain got to 5, Mrs. Wiley would use the PCA. Pain control better when nurse administered oral meds q3h instead of prn use of PCA.

Nursing Diagnoses	Clinical Outcomes	Interventions	Evaluation
		4. Review dose and meds for possible changes.	Pain 3–4 with ambulation at discharge.
		5. Teach relaxation techniques.	*M. E. Murray, RN 11/02/00*
		6. Encourage patient to use PCA before physical therapy (PT).	
Risk for caregiver role strain (upon discharge) related to dependency of frail spouse and surgery of caregiver	Caregiver and husband will identify needs at home and plan for assistance during care planning conference.	1. As part of discharge plan, discuss with patient, husband, and family who does what tasks in household. 2. Identify tasks Mrs. Wiley will be unable to complete for a time. 3. Clarify Mrs. Wiley's needs for rest and activity during rehab. 4. Problem solve additional sources of aid. 5. Communicate to the home health care agency selected by Mr. and Mrs. Wiley.	Outcome met. Family conference held and written plan developed to include home health nursing and Meals-on-Wheels. on temporary basis. *M. E. Murray, RN 11/02/00*
Impaired physical mobility, level 2*, related to knee replacement surgery	Patient will safely demonstrate independent ambulation and stair climbing with crutches by discharge.	1. Teach use of trapeze to assist movement. 2. Teach placement of crutches to facilitate getting out of bed, chair, up from toilet. 3. Teach upper-arm resistance exercises with 2- to 5-lb weight	Outcome partially met. Using trapeze and moving in bed. Crutch walking adequate. Still some confusion with crutch walking on stairs. Will continue PT in home and use walker. *M. E. Murray, RN 11/02/00*

* Requires help from another person for assistance, supervision, or teaching.

Nursing Diagnoses	Clinical Outcomes	Interventions	Evaluation
Risk for injury (Mrs. Wiley) related to lack of experience with crutch walking	Patient will remain free of falls during hospitaliza- tion and home recovery.	1. Premedicate 1 hour before physical therapy. 2. Physical therapist to reinstruct in crutch walking and transfers. 3. Supervised 2/day PT while in hospital. 4. Evaluate for at- home physical therapy upon discharge.	Outcome met during hospitalization; no falls have occurred. Mrs. Wiley is improv- ing in crutch walking and understands safety practices. Refer to home health agency for PT.

M. E. Murray, RN 11/02/00 |

EVALUATION #4
HOME HEALTH CARE AGENCY

Mrs. Wiley: Plan of care is designed by the nurse at the time of home health visit.

Nursing Diagnoses	Clinical Outcomes	Interventions	Evaluation
Knowledge/skill deficit: S/S to report to MD; aseptic technique; self- administered medication, purpose, schedule; wound care; pain management techniques	Reports elevated temperature/ chills to MD within 2 hours. Attains healing of wound without com- plications within 14 days. Demonstrates aseptic technique during wound care by second visit.	1. Teach S/S of infection to report to MD. 2. Teach aseptic technique for dressing changes. 3. Change dressing at incision site and instruct patient in assessment and process.	Outcome met. At second visit patient states, "I am comfort- able caring for myself now. It was so fast in the hospital, I couldn't take it all in. Now that I am home, it is so much easier." Incision dry, skin intact at 2-week check. Pt. states S/S of infec- tion, can change dressing using aseptic technique.

C. Hastert, RN 11/05/00 |

Nursing Diagnoses	Clinical Outcomes	Interventions	Evaluation
Acute pain related to joint replacement surgery, physical therapy, and movement	Maintains pain at 2 or less during week 1 at home.	1. Teach pain management techniques: relaxation, medication, cold application. 2. Alternate OTC meds and Tylenol #3. 3. Medicate 1 hour before PT.	Outcome met. At end of second visit, patient rates pain at 1–2. States, "I only take the Tylenol with codeine before PT, but I take the ibuprofen every 6 hours. That schedule seems to make the difference." *C. Hastert, RN 11/05/00*
Risk for injury (Mrs. Wiley) related to lack of experience with crutch walking	Remains free of falls at home.	1. Reinforce PT exercises. 2. Teach resistance exercises for upper-body strength, using soup cans for weights. 3. Assess home for hazards with each visit: wet floors, cluttered steps, home entrances. Suggest night-lights, steps, railings, grab bars. 4. Discuss winter weather precautions.	Outcome met. At termination of service to Mrs. Wiley, no falls have occurred. *C. Hastert, RN 11/05/00*

Bibliography

ALFARO-LEFEVRE, R. (1995). *Critical Thinking in Nursing: A Practical Approach*. Philadelphia, Saunders.

ALLIGOOD, M. and MARRINER-TOMEY, A. (1977). *Nursing Theory: Utilization and Application*. St. Louis, Mosby Year Book.

AMERICAN ASSOCIATION OF COLLEGES OF NURSING (1998). *The Essentials of Baccalaureate Education for Professional Nursing Practice*. Washington, D.C.

AMERICAN NURSES ASSOCIATION (1995). *Nursing's Social Policy Statement*. Washington, D.C., American Nurses Association.

AMERICAN NURSES ASSOCIATION (1998). *Managed Care: Nursing's Blueprint for Action*. Washington, D.C., American Nurses Association.

AMERICAN NURSES ASSOCIATION (1998). *Standards of Clinical Nursing Practice*, 2d ed. Washington, D.C., American Nurses Publishing, American Nurses Foundation/American Nurses Association.

ATKINSON, L., and MURRAY, M. E. (1995). *Clinical Guide to Care Planning: Data to Diagnosis*. New York, McGraw-Hill.

BANDMAN, E., and BANDMAN, B. (1995). *Critical Thinking in Nursing*, 2d ed. E. Norwalk, Conn., Appleton & Lange.

BENNER, P. (1984). *From Novice to Expert*. Menlo Park, Calif., Addison-Wesley.

BERGER, K., and WILLIAMS, M. (1999). *Fundamentals of Nursing: Collaborating For Optimum Health*, 2d ed. Stamford, Conn., Appleton & Lange.

BODENHEIMER, T., and GRUMBACH, K. (1998). *Understanding Health Policy: A Clinical Approach*, 2d ed. Stamford, Conn., Appleton & Lange.

BURRELL, L., GERLACH, M., and PLESS, B. (1997). *Foundations of Contemporary Nursing Practice*, 2d ed. Stamford, Conn., Appleton & Lange.

CENTER FOR HEALTH SCIENCES AT UNIVERSITY OF CALIFORNIA, SAN FRANCISCO (1997). Managed care and nursing: Is the sky really falling? *Front and Center* 2(1):1, 4, 7, 10.

DELAUNE, S., and LADNER, P. (1998). *Fundamentals of Nursing: Standards & Practice*. Albany, N.Y., Delmar.

FACIONE, N., FACIONE, P., and SANCHEZ, C. (1994). Critical thinking disposition as a measure of competent clinical judgement: The development of the

California critical thinking disposition inventory. *Journal of Nursing Education* 33(8):345–350.

FORKNER, J. (1996). Clinical pathways: Benefits and liabilities. *Nursing Management* 27(11):35–38.

GEISSLER, E. (1994). *Cultural Assessment.* St. Louis, Mosby.

GIGER, J. N., and DAVIDHIZAR, R. E. (1991). *Transcultural Nursing: Assessment and Intervention.* St. Louis, Mosby Year Book.

GREENWOOD, D. (1996). Nursing care plans: Issues and solutions. *Nursing Management* 27(3):33–40.

GREENWOOD, J., and KING, M. (1995). Some surprising similarities in the clinical reasoning of "expert" and "novice" orthopaedic nurses: Report of a study using verbal protocols and protocol analyses. *Journal of Advanced Science* 22:907–913.

HENDERSON, V. (1978). *The Nature of Nursing.* New York, Macmillan.

HUNT, R., and ZUREK, E. (1997). *Introduction to Community Based Nursing.* Philadelphia, Lippincott.

ITANO, J. (1989). A comparison of the clinical judgement process in experienced registered nurses and student nurses. *Journal of Nursing Education* 18(3):120–126.

JOHNSON, M., and MAAS, M., eds, (1997). *Nursing Outcomes Classification (NOC).* St. Louis, Mosby Year Book.

JOINT COMMISSION ON THE ACCREDITATION OF HEALTHCARE ORGANIZATIONS (1999.) *Hospital Accreditation Standards.* Chicago, JCAHO.

KATAOKA-YAHIRO, M., and SAYLOR, C. (1994). A critical thinking model for nursing judgement. *Journal of Nursing Education* 33(8):351–356.

KIRK, R. (1997). *Managing Outcomes, Process, and Cost in a Managed Care Environment.* Gaithersburg, Md., Aspen.

KOZIER, B., ERB, G., BLAIS, K., and WILKINSON, J. (1995). *Fundamentals of Nursing*, 5th ed. Redwood City, Calif., Addison-Wesley.

LEDDY, S. K. (1998). *Conceptual Bases of Professional Nursing.* Philadelphia, Lippincott.

LEE, P. R., and ESTES, C. L. (1997). *The Nation's Health*, 5th ed. Sudbury, Mass., Jones and Bartlett.

LEININGER, M. (1995). *Transcultural Nursing: Concepts, Theories, Research and Practice*, 2d ed. New York, McGraw-Hill.

LINDSET, E., and HARTRICK, G. (1996). Health-promoting nursing practice: The demise of the nursing process? *Journal of Advanced Nursing* 23:106–112.

MALONE, B., and MARULLO, G. (1997). *Workforce Trends among U.S. Registered Nurses*. American Nurses Association Policy Series, Washington, D.C., American Nurses Association.

MASLOW, A. (1968). *Toward a Psychology of Being*. New York, Van Nostrand.

MASON, G., and ATTREE, M. (1997). The relationship between research and the nursing process in clinical practice. *Journal of Advanced Nursing* 26:1045–1049.

MCCLOSKEY, J., and BULECHEK, G., eds. (1996). *Nursing Interventions Classification (NIC)*. 2d ed. St. Louis, Mosby Year Book.

MCFARLANE, M. (1998). Managed care: Nursing's friend or foe? *The Nursing Spectrum*, March 9, pp. 14–16.

MERRILL, E. (1998). Culturally diverse students enrolled in nursing: Barriers influencing success. *Journal of Cultural Diversity* 5(2):58–67.

MINNESOTA PUBLIC HEALTH ASSOCIATION'S IMMIGRANT HEALTH TASK FORCE (1996). *Six Steps toward Cultural Competence*. Minneapolis, Minnesota.

MORE, P., and MANDELL, S. (1997). *Nursing Case Management: An Evolving Practice*. New York, McGraw-Hill.

NATIONAL LEAGUE FOR NURSING (1989). *Criterion for the Evaluation of Baccalaureate and High Degree Programs in Nursing*, 6th ed. New York, National League for Nursing.

NORTH AMERICAN NURSING DIAGNOSIS ASSOCIATION (1999). *Nursing Diagnosis: Definitions and Classification 1999–2000*. Philadelphia, North American Nursing Diagnosis Association.

NURSING TRENDS & ISSUES (1998). *Nursing values challenged by managed care. Nursing Trends & Issues* 3(1):1–9.

OREM, D. E. (1985). *Nursing Concepts of Practice*. New York, McGraw-Hill.

PESUT, D., and HERMAN, J. (1998). OPT: Transformation of nursing process for contemporary practice. *Nursing Outlook* 46(1):29–36.

ROY, SISTER C. (1984). *Introduction to Nursing: An Adaptation Model*, 2d ed. Norwalk, Conn., Appleton-Century-Crofts.

SEDLAK, C., and LUDWICK R. (1996). Dressing up nursing diagnosis. *Nurse Educator* 21(4):19–22.

SIMPSON, K., LAVIN, M., and VEZEAU, T. (1998). Second opinion: Is there a future for nursing diagnosis? *Maternal-Child Nursing Journal* 23(6):290–291.

SMELTZER, S., and BARE, B. (1996). *Brunner and Suddarth's Textbook of Medical-Surgical Nursing*, 8th ed. Philadelphia, Lippincott.

SPECTOR, R. E. (1991). *Cultural Diversity in Health and Illness*, 3d ed. Norwalk, Conn., Appleton & Lange.

SWANSBURG, R. C., and SWANSBURG, R. J. (1999). *Introductory Management and Leadership for Nurses*, 2d ed. Subdury, Mass., Jones and Bartlett.

TURNER, S. O. (1999). *The Nurse's Guide to Managed Care*. Gaithersburg, Md., Aspen.

VARCOE, C. (1996). Disparagement of the nursing process: The new dogma? *Journal of Advanced Nursing* 23:120–125.

YODER-WISE, P. (1999). *Leading and Managing in Nursing*, 2d ed. St. Louis, Mosby.

ZANDER, K. (1992). Quantifying, managing and improving quality. *The New Definition* 7(4):1–4.

Sample Nursing Care Plans

NURSING CARE PLAN #1. MIDDLE ADULT

Lyman, John
66550250
Dr. Burns/Snyder
Room 231 55 yrs

NURSING ASSESSMENT

(Data Collection Format based on the Functional Health Patterns developed by Gordon, 1982)

General Information

Information given by: patient

Name: Mr. John Lyman

Age: 55 yrs   Sex: male   Race: Caucasian

Admission date/time: 7/6/00; 2100 hours

Admitting medical diagnosis: "possible heart attack"

Arrived on unit by: wheelchair   from: home

Accompanied by: daughter

Admitting weight/VS: 188 lbs, 5'11"; T. 99.0, P. 96, R. 28, BP 120/70

Allergies: no known allergies

Medications: no prescription meds

NURSING CARE PLAN #1 (CONT.)

Health Perception–Health Management

Patient's perception of reason for admission: <u>severe pain in middle of chest,</u>
<u>upper abdomen region; "the doctor thinks I might have had a heart attack;</u>
<u>I've never had anything like this before"</u>
How has problem been managed by patient at home? <u>"I sat down and tried to</u>
<u>relax, then I lay down, but nothing helped; the chest pain just kept getting worse,</u>
<u>so I called the doctor and she said to come right in"</u>

Nutritional–Metabolic Pattern

states he is about 15 lbs overweight; eats 2–3 meals a day, often skips breakfast; cooks for himself but eats out frequently; reports alcohol consumption of 2–3 drinks/week

SKIN: mucous membranes pink; good skin turgor; diaphoretic, pale

LAST INTAKE: at 6 P.M. ate a pizza; denies any nausea on admission

FOOD ALLERGIES: none

Elimination Pattern

BOWEL: last BM on 7/6; usual pattern qd; denies taking laxatives/softeners; bowel sounds present in all 4 quadrants

URINARY: denies any changes in urinary elimination patterns; no difficulty initiating; voids in large amounts, no burning; last voiding on admission to hospital—states it was normal large amount

EDEMA: no edema noted in ankles or fingers; denies any problems with edema; ring is not tight

Activity–Exercise Pattern

no physical limitations; reports going to the health club 2–3 times a week for weight machines and occasional racquetball games; no daily exercise program

RESPIRATORY: reports slight dyspnea; some diaphoresis noted; respirations nonlabored but slightly deeper and more rapid than normal; lung sounds clear;

no cyanosis noted on admission; smokes 2 packs/day; reports he has tried to quit twice but really enjoys smoking and lives alone, so no one complains

CARDIAC: normal BP 150/90; 120/70 on admission; pulse rapid, strong radial pulse, 96/min and irregular; reports feeling occasional palpitations for last hour; monitor shows normal sinus rhythm, occasional PVCs (1–4/min) over 15 minutes since admission

Sleep–Rest Pattern

6 hours a night is normal pattern; denies use of sleeping medications

Cognitive–Perceptual Pattern

PAIN: states he was watching TV when the pain started in the midchest area; described as viselike and radiated down left arm; "pain got worse and worse over about an hour"; rated as 8 on 1–10 scale

ANALGESICS: states he has taken nothing for pain but really needs something now

SENSES: denies any hearing, speech, or visual problems; states he probably needs glasses because things are getting blurry up as close as he used to hold them; denies any changes in sensation, no numbness of fingers/toes

ORIENTATION: oriented to time, place, and person; states he feels "just awful" and is afraid he is going to die

Self-Perception–Self-Concept Pattern

reports being afraid of dying or being a burden to his family; "my father died of a heart attack in his fifties" and "I have had high blood pressure and an elevated cholesterol for 3 years that I know of"; three married daughters; one lives in town and brought him in; divorced 4 years ago from his wife of 25 years; lives alone and states he is very independent; "couldn't live with my daughters and have them take care of me"; reports he works hard and long hours as a financial adviser; "my daughters have been after me to take it easier and take some time off, but I just never seem to find the time"

Role–Relationship Pattern

lives alone since divorce 4 years ago; ex-wife out of state and does not want her notified of his condition; three married daughters; visits the one in town every few weeks and occasionally baby-sits his grandchildren

Sexuality–Reproductive Pattern

vasectomy 1979; reports no problems with sexual part of his life; "I've kind of been on hold since the divorce; I suppose I won't have to worry about that anymore, though; if this is a heart attack, I know sex is out for me"

Coping–Stress Tolerance Pattern

"I guess I am under a lot of stress at work; the stock market is hard to predict, but my clients expect me to always make a profit; sometimes I feel like every one is pulling on me to do things for them; I'm going to have to make a few phone calls to work. How do I get an outside line?"

Value–Belief Pattern

Catholic; attends church every week; reports he would like to see his priest if he gets worse

Priority Nursing Diagnoses	Outcomes
1. Fear related to possible myocardial infarction (MI) and risk of dying as manifested by own statements, elevated pulse and respirations	Reduction in fear reported; identification of methods of coping with/reducing fear of MI/dying/reoccurrence by disch. ∘ states feeling less fearful in 1 hour ∘ states understanding of tests, treatments before implementing ∘ states understanding of risk factors in life-style and changes needed to reduce risk by discharge ∘ identifies support system to decrease fears within 1 hour
2. Pain related to possible myocardial hypoxia as manifested by rating pain an 8, elevated pulse and diaphoresis	Report of negligible pain by discharge ∘ pain reported at a level of 3 or less within the next hour with the use of oxygen and nitro-glycerin. ∘ pain maintained at a level of 3 or less during the next 48 hours with analgesics

MIDDLE ADULT (CONT.)

Priority Nursing Diagnoses	Outcomes
3. High risk for decreased cardiac output related to inadequate pumping of the heart secondary to possible MI	Maintains adequate tissue perfusion during hospitalization ◦ maintains clear lung sounds during next 48 hours ◦ presence of strong peripheral pulses during next 48 hours ◦ maintains heart rate at 70–100 with no cyanosis while hospitalized

Nursing Interventions	Rationale
1. a. Assess understanding and teach prn before tests, tx., interventions.	a. Provides baseline data from which to teach; begin at learner's level of understanding; knowing what to expect decreases fear.
b. Offer opportunity to share fears, concerns q4h × 24h; reassure realistically; point out positive sign of status/ functioning.	b. Identifying and discussing fears give nurse a chance to understand and support without giving false reassurance; focus on positive gives encouragement and hope.
c. Encourage daughter to stay.	c. Presence of support people can decrease fear, increase feelings of safety/security.
d. Have patient/family write down their questions for the doctor or nurse.	d. Unanswered questions/ confusion can cause concern; patients often forget to ask questions when MD or nurse in room.
e. Orient to room, all equipment.	e. Unfamiliar environment can cause anxiety/fear.
f. Offer to contact hospital chaplain anytime patient desires.	f. Meeting spiritual needs can decrease anxiety and give hope; opportunity to express concerns.
g. Assign consistent nursing personnel whenever possible: Adams, Grahm, Tran.	g. Development of trusting therapeutic relationship decreases fear.
h. Involve in planning own care; explain how he can maximize medical and nursing treatment to promote recovery.	h. Give sense of control, which can decrease fear; promotes cooperation with treatments.

NURSING CARE PLAN #1 (CONT.)

Nursing Interventions	Rationale

i. When physical status stabilizes
  ◦ assess knowledge of heart disease and risk factors in his life
  ◦ provide information as needed
  ◦ work with him on ways to reduce risk factors and attain maximum recovery
  ◦ discuss possibility of family conference involving daughters, doctor, nurses for discussion of life-style changes; medical management of condition; abilities, limitations, schedule for resumption of activities and work responsibilities
  ◦ identify community resources/ groups that pt. may join
	i. Readiness to learn life-style changes begins with recovery phase of illness; input and support from all involved result in more realistic plan, increased commitment to plan.

2. a. Assess knowledge of reason for pain and assessments; explain as needed to patient/family.	a. Teaching begins at the learner's level of understanding to be most effective; understanding cause of pain makes tx. more understandable.

b. Assess vital signs and pain; begin O$_2$, nitroglycerin per doctor's order
  ◦ begin morphine IV per doctor's order if O$_2$ and nitroglycerin not effective
  ◦ respirations, pulse and BP qh
  ◦ level of consciousness qh
  ◦ notify MD if R>14, BP>100/70
  ◦ assess and reassure during first 15 min of morphine administration if needed
  ◦ side rail up
	b. Provides baseline data from which response to treatment is judged
	
	  ◦ morphine can depress respirations
	  ◦ morphine causes vasodilation and possible hypotensive response
	  ◦ morphine can cause euphoric state; dizziness or fainting can occur if patient tries to stand

MIDDLE ADULT (CONT.)

Nursing Interventions	Rationale
c. Oxygen per doctor's order; assess concentration, response qh.	c. Morphine may depress respirations; increasing amount of oxygen to heart tissue will help reduce pain.
d. Position in semi-Fowler's position (head or bed up at 45 degrees).	d. Generally more comfortable position if SOB; lowers diaphragm and increases lung expansion.
e. Explain and implement bed rest order; place urinal, phone, water within reach.	e. Decreases work load on heart and oxygen requirements; may decrease pain.
f. Environmental management to promote rest.	f. Noisy, bright room with many people talking and doing things interferes with ability to rest and produces added stress/anxiety.
g. Offer techniques to promote relaxation/pain management.	g. Decreased muscle tension reduces oxygen needs of muscles; distraction, imagery can reduce perception of pain and promote rest.
3. a. Assess per doctor's order and report significant changes to physician in areas of ◦ vital signs qh ◦ urine volume q2h or q voiding ◦ skin temp/peripheral pulses ◦ lung sounds ◦ regularity of heartbeat	a. Assessment data provide baseline for comparison of changes that may indicate changing condition and need for adjustment of nursing and medical treatment plan ◦ decreased urine output may indicate inadequate blood flow to kidney, dehydration ◦ deterioration in pumping action of heart can lead to dropping BP, increased or decreased heart rate, increase in PVCs, cold pale skin and weak or absent pulses in extremities, buildup of fluid in lungs with moist breath sounds developing.
b. Oxygen per doctor's order; assess concentration, response qh (explain "no smoking" rule).	b. Increased oxygen content of inspired air provides more oxygen to all body tissues; oxygen promotes burning, and smoking could cause a fire.

NURSING CARE PLAN #1 (CONT.)

Nursing Interventions	Rationale
c. Assist with position changes q2h (head of bed up at 45 degrees).	c. Alternating pressure areas will promote adequate circulation and oxygenation of weight-bearing body tissues.
d. Explain and implement bed rest order; place urinal, phone, water within reach.	d. Decreases work load on heart and improves circulation to legs.
e. Accurate intake-output recordings and daily weights.	e. Dehydration can decrease the circulating blood volume, resulting in decreased perfusion of periphery; excess fluid can cause accumulation in the lungs; maintenance of normal weight reflects adequate hydration and no fluid retention.

CRITICAL/CLINICAL PATHWAY—CHF (CONGESTIVE HEART FAILURE)

Lyman, John
66550250
Dr. Burns/Snyder
Room 231 55 yrs

CHF Care Management Model Outcomes Guide

Inclusion Criteria	Exclusion Criteria	
Primary Diagnosis CHF	Secondary Diagnosis of CHF Pulmonary Edema Renal Failure	Acute MI Unstable Angina

*Refer to Variance Note

Patient/Family Outcomes   Review Daily

Care Category	Desired Outcomes	Met (Date/ Initial)	Not Met* (Date/ Initial)
Disease Process	Verbalizes symptoms of heart failure		
Physical Assessment	_ _ Class I: No activity limitations or symptoms. _ _ Class II: Moderate limitation, dyspnea with exertion. _ _ Class III: Marked limitation, dyspnea with minimal exertion. _ _ Class IV: Severe limitation, inability to carry on activities.		

MIDDLE ADULT (CONT.)

Care Category	Desired Outcomes	Met	Not Met*
Activity	Verbalizes understanding of activity within physical limitations Describes energy-sparing plans		
Nutrition	Verbalizes understanding of salt restriction Verbalizes understanding of fluid restriction Describes prescribed dietary and fluid intake plan		
Medications	Verbalizes understanding of purpose of prescribed medications Describes appearance of prescribed medications Demonstrates use of medication schedule Verbalizes understanding of not using nonprescription drugs		
Monitoring	Verbalizes understanding of monitoring daily weight Demonstrates recording daily weight Describes signs/symptoms of fluid retention Verbalizes understanding of when to contact clinic Verbalizes understanding of when to go to emergency department		
Spiritual	Verbalizes end-of-life concerns Expresses needs relating to faith and/or belief system Expresses concerns relating to interactions with others		
Discharge	Describes postdischarge plan of care States understanding of information provided		

Patient Educator Referral Criteria
Patient and/or family members who:
* Appear anxious or express unusual anxiety related to diagnosis/disease process/treatment plan
* Are unable to read or have sensory impairments
* Do not learn well with the methods provided
* Have identified barriers to learning (language, cultural, emotional, physical, cognitive, spiritual)
* Have unanswered questions that nursing staff is unable to address
* Primary or new diagnosis of CHF
To contact cardiovascular patient educator call 520-5054

Activity Level

Activity Level	Description
0	Independent
1	Minimal limitation
2	Requires assistive device (list): _ _ _ _ _ _ _ _ _ _ _ _ _
3	Requires assistance/supervision of another
4	Requires assistance of another and use of assistive device
5	Dependent, unable to participate in activity

Initials	Signatures	Initials	Signatures	Initials	Signatures

Lyman, John
66550250
Dr. Burns/Snyder
Room 231   55 yrs

CHF Care Model

Admission 7/6/00	Date 7/7/00	Date 7/8/00	Date 7/9/00
Diagnostics	**Diagnostics**	**Diagnostics**	**Diagnostics**
Lytes ✓ BUN ✓ Creat ✓ Glucose ✓ Dig level __ CXR __, EKG ✓ Echo (if none in 6 mo.)	(if not done in ED) K + WNL __ __ __ __ Coag studies __ __ __ __	K + WNL __ __ __ __	K + WNL __ __ __ __
Activity	**Activity**	**Activity**	**Activity**
Bed rest ✓ Bedside commode ✓ BRPs __ __ __ __ __ Tolerates ordered activity Y __ N __	Cardiac rehab activity assessment Y __ N __ (Order # __ __) Up ad lib Y __ N __ Ordered activity __ __ __ Met ( ) Not met ( ) Pt/family review importance of balancing activity/rest Y __ N __	Ordered activity __ __ __ __ Met ( ) Not met ( ) Up ad lib Y __ N __ Tolerates activity Y __ N __ Pt/family review importance of exercise Y __ N __	Ordered activity __ __ __ __ Met ( ) Not met ( ) Up ad lib Y __ N __ Tolerates activity Y __ N __ Pt/family review plan for regular activity/exercise plan Y __ N __
Nutrition	**Nutrition**	**Nutrition**	**Nutrition**
2 g Sodium restriction Y __ N ✓ Fluid restriction __ ml Fluid per shift 7-3 __ 3-11 __ 11-7 __ __ *RD ref. CHF Adm. Y __ N __ Order # __	2 g Sodium restriction Y __ N ✓ Fluid restriction __ ml/day Fluid per shift 7-3 __ 3-11 __ 11-7 __ __ *RD assess nutrition status Y __ N __	2 g Sodium restriction Y __ N __ Fluid restriction __ ml/day Fluid per shift 7-3 __ 3-11 __ 11-7 __ __ *RD sodium assess Y __ N __	2 g Sodium restriction Y __ N __ Fluid restriction __ ml/day Fluid per shift 7-3 __ 3-11 __ 11-7 __ __ *Pt/family review recommended nutrition/fluid plan Y __ N __
Treatments/Interventions	**Treatments/Interventions**	**Treatments/Interventions**	**Treatments/Interventions**
IV fluid D5 1/2 NS5 75k Saline lock __ Oxygen 2-3 l/min Oximetry q 1 h	IV fluid __ DC? __ Saline lock __ Oxygen __ DC? __ Oximetry __ DC? __	IV fluid __ DC? __ Saline lock __ Oxygen __ DC? __ Oximetry __ DC? __	IV fluid __ DC? __ Saline lock __ DC? __ Oxygen __ DC? __ Oximetry __ DC? __

I and O ____✓____ Daily weight ____✓____ Telemetry ____✓____ Foley catheter ________	I and O ________ Daily weight ________ Telemetry ________ Foley catheter ____ DC? ____	I and O ________ Daily weight ________ Telemetry ____ DC? ____ Foley catheter ____ DC? ____	I and O ________ Daily weight ________ Telemetry ____ DC? ____ Foley catheter ____ DC? ____
Signs and Symptoms WNL Breath sounds Y ✓ N _ Work of breathing Y ✓ N _ Peripheral edema Y ✓ N _ Vital signs Y _ N ✓ Cardiac rhythm Y _ N ✓	***Signs and Symptoms WNL*** Breath sounds Y _ N _ Work of breathing Y _ N _ Peripheral edema Y _ N _ Vital signs Y _ N _ Cardiac rhythm Y _ N _	***Signs and Symptoms WNL*** Breath sounds Y _ N _ Work of breathing Y _ N _ Peripheral edema Y _ N _ Vital signs Y _ N _ Cardiac rhythm Y _ N _	***Signs and Symptoms WNL*** Breath sounds Y _ N _ Work of breathing Y _ N _ Peripheral edema Y _ N _ Vital signs Y _ N _ Cardiac rhythm Y _ N _
Discharge Planning DPQ completed ___ Blaylock completed ___ Interdisciplinary referral form completed? Y _ N _ Patient education packet provided Y _ N _	***Discharge Planning*** D/C planning group Y _ N _ Referral to cardiovascular patient educator? Y _ N _ NA _ Home care needs: Scale Y _ N _ 02 Y _ N _ Home health referral Y _ N _ Social service referral Y _ N _	***Discharge Planning*** D/C planning group Y _ N _ Instruct pt regarding: Record daily weight Y _ N _ Signs of exacerbation Y _ N _ When to call MD/911 Y _ N _	***Discharge Planning*** CHF follow-up visit _ _ _ _ _ _ _ _ Home health referral Y _ N _ Patient education packet Y _ N _ Scale: Has _ Sent with pt. _
Self-Care Management Plan Learning barriers? Y _ N ✓ List ________ Review disease process and reason for admission with pt/family Y _ N _ Provide med. info Y _ N _	***Self-Care Management Plan*** Pt/family view/review: CHF video Y _ N _ Prewritten D/C instructions Y _ N _ Daily weight record Y _ N _ Medications Y _ N _ Modifiable risk factors Y _ N _	***Self-Care Management Plan*** Pt/family to review: Signs and symptoms to report to MD/NP/911 Y _ N _ Self-record daily weight Y _ N _ Medication: Schedule Y _ N _ Dose Y _ N _ Common side effects Y _ N _	***Teaching Plan*** Pt/family review discharge plan related to: Diet Y _ N _ Daily weight log Y _ N _ Activity/rest Y _ N _ Medications Y _ N _ Symptoms to report Y _ N _
Medications Ace inhibitor Y _ N _ Beta blocker Y _ N _ Diuretic Y _ N _ Anticoagulant Y ✓ N _ K+ Y ✓ N _ MG++ Y _ N _	***Medications*** Ace inhibitor Y _ N _ Beta blocker Y _ N _ Diuretic Y _ N _ Anticoagulant Y _ N _ K+ Y _ N _ MG++ Y _ N _	***Medications*** Ace inhibitor Y _ N _ Beta blocker Y _ N _ Diuretic Y _ N _ Anticoagulant Y _ N _ K+ Y _ N _ MG++ Y _ N _	***Medications*** Ace inhibitor Y _ N _ Beta blocker Y _ N _ Diuretic Y _ N _ Anticoagulant Y _ N _ K+ Y _ N _ MG++ Y __ N __

Nursing Care Plan #2, Senior Adult

By Tom Olson, PhD, RN

Harada, Fred
89645412
Dr. Sharp/Johnson
Progressive Care Facility, Room 109
78 yrs

NURSING ASSESSMENT

(Data Collection Format adapted from Human Response Patterns described by NANDA, 1999)

General Information

Information given by: client and son

Name: Mr. Fred Harada

Age: 78 yrs   Sex: male

Ethnicity/race: Japanese-American (Nisei—2d generation)

Admission date/time: 2/1/00

Arrived on unit: ambulatory

Accompanied by: son

Admitting medical diagnosis: inability to care for self at home; weight loss;

mild hypertension history; short-term memory deficit; R/O major

depression and/or dementia

Admitting weight/VS: 140 lbs, 5'7"; T, 97.0, P. 90, R. 20, BP 140/88,

no c/o pain

Client's perception of reason for admission: "I was fine until my wife died.

Now I'm just tired, and I don't see much purpose in anything, including

being here. My son probably told you that I haven't been eating. I'm just

not hungry. Please leave me alone"

How had problems been managed at home? son visits weekly but reports

father increasingly difficult to engage in conversation; has lost contact

SENIOR ADULT (CONT.)

with friends, appears disheveled, forgets recent events, refuses to eat and

"continues to lose weight"

Allergies: no known allergies

Medications: "something for my blood pressure" (Inderal)

Exchanging

NUTRITION: wears dentures, states they do not hurt, lips are pink but dry; poor skin turgor; appears gaunt, thin; reports normal smell but decreased taste of food; reports poor appetite; cooks for self; "food just doesn't taste good anymore"; son states father does not eat, won't shop for groceries; has lost 9 lbs in last 2 months

ELIMINATION: continent of bowel and bladder; denies taking laxatives; states normal pattern qd; denies trouble initiating or maintaining urination; voids large amounts several times a day; gets up at night 2 times to urinate

CIRCULATION: heart rate 90 and regular; strong pulses; BP 140/88 on admission; son states it used to be higher and father put on medication several years ago; feet and hands pale and cool

OXYGENATION: breath sounds clear; rate 20/minute; nonlabored; denies smoking; son says he quit 15 years ago; denies any difficulty breathing; son says lately his father tires easily and breathes harder with activity

PHYSICAL INTEGRITY: skin intact, dry; mucous membranes intact; no open sores; son states that father was not bathing, shaving, or doing personal hygiene; nails dirty, slight odor

Communication

does not initiate conversation; responds to direct questions with brief answers; shoulders slumped, head down with minimal eye contact; denies any hearing problem; speech not impaired

Relating

SOCIALIZATION: son states father used to be outgoing and was active with his wife in church and around the house; son states father has progressively withdrawn from contact and communication since wife's death 8 months ago

NURSING CARE PLAN #2 (CONT.)

ROLE: son states his father was a carpenter who remained active with projects after retirement but now doesn't do anything; doesn't call family or relate to grandchildren when visiting; patient states, "I've got nothing to do; no point in doing anything anymore"; denies having any close friends, "they are all dead or put away"; says son busy with his own life and doesn't have time for him (son lives out of town, 1 hour away; client's only child)

Valuing

states that he used to go to church with his wife every Sunday but did it for her, so now there is no point going; repeatedly states that he sees "no point" or purpose in life situation

Choosing

COPING: "I just don't care anymore"; reports thinking about wife frequently; son reports his father is having increasing difficulty making even simple decisions, so leaves bills, shopping, cooking, and similar tasks unattended; son adds, "I'm not sure to what extent he's unable to care for himself or just unwilling"

Moving

MOBILITY–ACTIVITY: son reports father tires more easily since he has lost weight; "stopped caring about himself"; no physical limitations; no activities except watching TV; gait is steady but very slow

REST–SLEEP: client states tired all the time; difficulty both initiating sleep and remaining asleep—awakens 3–4 times per night with 4–5 hours of sleep; naps frequently during the day; son states that his father is always sleeping in a chair when he visits

ACTIVITIES OF DAILY LIVING: son states he does not think that his father is able to live alone and manage for himself in his present situation (see also exchanging/physical integrity and choosing/coping)

Perceiving

SELF-CONCEPT: states he is "useless"; feels "helpless without his wife"; no good to anyone anymore

SENSORY–PERCEPTION: no changes in sensation; wears bifocals; states he hears well

Knowing–Thought Processes

no evidence of altered thought process; sentences logical, appropriate responses; oriented to time, place, and person; son reports that his father "forgets that I've called or visited him"; long-term memory intact

Feeling

COMFORT: denies any pain; "stiff sometimes"

EMOTIONAL STATES–INTEGRITY: "everything takes so much effort since my wife died. I can't stop thinking about her. I wish it had been me. It's hard to be the one left"; denies feeling suicidal: "that's wrong"; minimal change in facial expression and tone of voice (see also data under communication); frequent sighing

Priority Nursing Diagnoses	Outcomes	Nursing Interventions	Rationale
Altered nutrition: less than body requirements related to lack of interest in food as evidenced by 9-lb weight loss	Weight will stabilize at his previous level of 149 lbs within 3 months. Evaluate 5/1. • Report of appetite returning during the next week. Evaluate 2/8.	1. Observe, record, report I&O. 2. Weigh q A.M. 3. Assess food preferences. 4. Assist in filling out daily menu.	1. Monitor client's progress/evaluate effectiveness of plan. 2. As above. 3. Taking into account client's likes/dislikes may stimulate appetite. 4. Involve client in plan to increase cooperation. Ensure nutritionally balanced meal.
	• Weight gain of 3 lbs at end of 2 weeks. Evaluate 2/15.	5. Consult with physician and dietitian re between-meal snacks, high-protein food supplenents, possible vitamin supplements. 6. Assist client with hygiene before meals.	5. Meet nutritional needs of client. 6. Increase psychological and physical readiness to eat.

NURSING CARE PLAN #2 (CONT.)

Priority Nursing Diagnoses	Outcomes	Nursing Interventions	Rationale
		7. Encourage client to sit with others in the dining room at mealtimes.	7. Normal eating situation tends to stimulate appetite.
Sleep pattern disturbances related to loss of wife, altered daytime activity pattern, frequent naps as evidenced by statements of inability to get to sleep, awakening 3–4 times per night, being tired all the time, difficulty initiating and sustaining sleep	Sleeping 6 hours through the night and decreased nighttime awakening to 2 or less during stay in nursing home.	1. Obtain a sleep history on pattern before the death of his wife and changes since death. 2. Assess for factors in nursing home environment that might interfere with sleep and try to minimize if possible. 3. Increase daytime activity: • dining room for meals • shower/bath daily— client choice • walk on grounds/in building for 15 minutes qid • encourage participation in group excercise session/activities 4. Offer back rub at HS. 5. Encourage good sleep hygiene • no caffeine after noon meal • limit cigarette smoking	1. Provides baseline data from which to assess activities that promote or interfere with sleep. 2. Noise, heat, cold, too hard or soft a bed, roommates, lights can all interfere with sleep. 3. Promote normal circadian rhythm. 4. Back rubs help relax muscles and give client time to talk about any concerns; relaxation and de-creased anxiety facilitate sleep. • caffeine is a stimulant • nicotine can stimulate CNS

SENIOR ADULT (CONT.)

Priority Nursing Diagnoses	Outcomes	Nursing Interventions	Rationale
		• offer light snack before bed	• foods high in protein and L-triptophan (milk) promote sleep
		• help to follow usual routine for hygiene, time	• normal habits from home associated with a good sleeping pattern
Dysfunctional grieving related to death of spouse as manifested by report of constantly thinking about his wife, blunted affect, self-imposed social isolation, physical neglect of self	Reestablished previous level of self-care, productivity, social contacts by 3/1. • expresses feelings related to loss of spouse within 1 week • identifies losses/ changes in his life because of wife's death by 2d week • identifies 2 adaptive ways of viewing his loss • independently reestablishes previous level of personal grooming by 4 weeks	1. Assess the existence, extent, and impact of unresolved losses through use of open-ended and direct questions; assess previous life patterns in expressing feelings. 2. Monitor any changes in memory or cognitive functions— use Mini-Mental Status Exam (MMSE) and Geriatric Depression scale. 3. Encourage client to verbalize feelings regarding losses. 4. Share own observations of client's behavior and seek clarification and confirmation. 5. Provide consistent caregiver.	1. Must assess types of unresolved losses and importance to client in order to fully implement plan. (Note: Elderly frequently have multiple unresolved losses.) 2. Assist in distinguishing between dysfunctional grieving/ depression and possible symptoms of dementia. 3. Increase data base; assist client in developing an awareness of predominant feelings. 4. As above. 5. Build rapport; develop trust.

NURSING CARE PLAN #2 (CONT.)

Priority Nursing Diagnoses	Outcomes	Nursing Interventions	Rationale
		6. Spend 10 minutes sitting with client bid; use touch as appropriate; remain with client despite lack of ability to verbalize.	6. Convey uncon- ditional acceptance so that client is free to express feelings.
		7. Look over the daily activity calendar with the client and leave a copy in his room; specifically suggest choosing one activity.	7. Involve client to improve coopera- tion. Individualize plan to ensure its likelihood of success. Decrease isolation.
		8. Encourage the client to sit with others in the dining room at mealtimes.	8. Gradually "repeople" client's life; supply opportuni- ties for develop- ment of meaning- ful relationships without over- whelming him. Reinforce sense of belonging.
		9. Introduce client to other residents on other units.	9. As above.
Situational low self-esteem related to loss of spouse and husband role as evidenced by expressions of hopelessness, uselessness, inability to do anything productive	Evaluate self as needed and competent by 3 months. • one positive statement of self-worth within 48 hours • begins work on one carpentry project by 2 weeks	1. Assess client's interests through the use of open-ended and direct questions and tool such as pleasant events schedule.	1. Necessary to guide plan.
		2. Assess for religious and spiritual beliefs and offer to accompany to services if desired.	2. Facilitate source of support.
		3. Encourage client to verbalize about	3. Continue assess- ment. Convey

SENIOR ADULT (CONT.)

Priority Nursing Diagnoses	Outcomes	Nursing Interventions	Rationale
		himself, especially his present feelings.	acceptance of client. Increase client awareness of feelings.
		4. Continue nursing actions 4–6 for Dysfunctional Grieving diagnosis above.	4. Same as 4–6 above.
		5. Maximize choices client can make.	5–7. Rebuild self-esteem.
		6. Assist with grooming as needed.	
		7. Give merited praise and recognition based on specific, accurate observation.	
		8. Occupational therapy referral for projects, needs of facility in carpentry.	8. Projects useful to facility in field of expertise reinforce usefulness, positive self-worth.
High risk for self-directed violence related to negative self-esteem and depression as evidenced by statements of wanting to be with dead wife, wishing that it had been he who died	Client will deny suicidal plans or ideas throughout stay in nursing home. Evaluate Friday of each week.	1. Directly ask the client if he is currently suicidal and systematically assess other self-harm factors including attempt history, plan, lethality of plan, access to plan, and anger.	1. Determine immediate need for intervention.
		2. Make verbal agreement with client that he will notify nursing staff if feeling out of control or suicidal.	2. Involve client in plan to ensure its success.
		3. If client feels suicidal, implement appropriate safety measures, such as moving client closer to nurses'	3. Increase nurse's accessibility to client and increase opportunities for

NURSING CARE PLAN #2 (CONT.)

Priority Nursing Diagnoses	Outcomes	Nursing Interventions	Rationale
		station, checking room for any items with which client might harm self, increase frequency of room checks, notify physician.	observation.
		4. Increase frequency of room checks to q 15 min.	4. Prevent, interfere with, or interrupt any self-destructive behavior.
		5. Monitor client behavior and observe especially for changes in mood or level of energy (be aware of greater risk after these changes).	5. Provide data with which to evaluate suicide potential; changes may signal increased suicide risk.
		6. Alert all staff regarding client's suicidal potential.	6. Provide safety and security for client.
		7. Spend 10 minutes sitting with client bid. Use touch as appropriate; remain with client despite lack of verbalization.	7. Build rapport; develop trust. Convey unconditional acceptance so client is free to express feelings.
		8. Permit verbalization of suicidal feelings; do not ignore them or argue with the client about them.	8. Establish trust. Recognize importance of intent.
		9. Carefully document client behavior and nursing actions.	9. Ensure consistency of care.

APPENDIX B

Web Sites

GENERAL NURSING WEB SITES

American Nurses Association   http://www.nursingworld.org

Joint Commission on Accreditation of Healthcare Organizations
http://www.jcaho.org/mainmenu.htm

Medicaid   http://www.hcfa.gov

Medicare   (same as above)

North American Nursing Diagnosis Association: E-mail
nanda@nursecominc.com

National Committee for Quality Assurance   http://www.ncqa.org/pages/main/index.htm

Nursing Interventions Classification   http://www.nursing.uiowa.edu/nic

Nursing Outcomes Classification   http://www.nursing.uiowa.edu/noc

GENERAL CULTURAL WEB SITES

http://www.hotbot.com

http://home.miningco.com/culture/cultureworld

http://www.altavista.com

http://www.about.com

SPECIFIC CULTURAL REFERENCES

African   Culture   http://afroamculture.about.com/index.htm?cob=home&pid=2744

Asia and the Pacific   http://www.asiasociety.org

http://asianamculture.miningco.com

Buddhism   http://www.kagyu.org

Chinese Culture   http://chineseculture.miningco.com
http://www.pavilion.co.uk/jcm/

http://www.healthy.net/pan/pa/acupuncture/naoma/
naoma.htm

http://www.qi-journal.com

English Culture   http://englishculture.miningco.com

French Culture   http://frenchculture.miningco.com

German Culture   http://germanculture.miningco.com

Greek Culture   http://velox.stanford.edu/hellas

http://www.hellenicweb.com

Hmong Culture   http://www.uwsp.edu

http://www.laofamily.org/hmongculture.htm

http://www.hotbot.com

http://www.hmongnet.org

Indian Culture   http://indianculture.miningco.com

http://indiafocus.indiainfo.com

http://india-site.net/isn/society/index.html

Israeli Culture   http://israeliculture.miningco.com

Italian Culture   http://italianculture.miningco.com

Japanese Culture   http://japaneseculture.miningco.com

Polish Culture   http://www.ampolinstitute.org/history.html

Russian Culture   http://valley.net/~transnat

http://russianculture.miningco.com

Scottish Culture   http://scottishculture.miningco.com

Somalian Culture   http://www.somali.com
                    http://www.arab.net/somali/culture/somalisab.html

Spanish Culture   http://spanishculture.miningco.com

Thai Culture   http://www.mahidol.ac.th/thailand/glance-thai/land.html
                http://www.frangipani.com/huahin/tips.htm

Index

Page numbers followed by *t* refer to tables; page numbers followed by *f* refer to figures.

A

Accountability, fiscal, 22
  Strategies for, 24
Action, nursing, 127
Activities of daily living (ADLs), 151
Activity-exercise pattern, on care plan, 212–213
Adaptation model, 31
AIDS patients, confidentiality and, 53
Alligood, M., 31
American Nurses Association (ANA), 1
  elements of nursing practice, 1–2
  nursing, definition of, 1
  on nursing diagnoses, 65, 69, 84
  Standards of Clinical Nursing Practice of, 6–7, 25, 65, 99, 127, 148, 159, 183
  web site for, 231
Appropriateness, of care plan, 160
Assessment, nursing, 2, 25
  American Nurses' Association standard of, 25
  on care plan, 211–214
  case studies, 56–63
    preop clinic 57–59
    first day surgery 59–60
    postop unit, 61
    home health agency, 61–63
  activities of, 26
  critical thinking for, 43–44
    prompts for, 44
  culturally competent care during, 48–51
    prompts for, 49–50
  data collection in, 26–42
  defined, 25

examples of, 43, 57–63, 211–214, 222–225
  managed care environment, 51–54
  practice exercises, 54–56
  reassessment, 189
  Skills for 33–42
Assessment framework
  Gordon's functional health patterns, 30, 211–214
  growth and development, 31–33
  Henderson's, 29–30
  Maslow's basic needs, 27
  NANDA's, 30, 222–225
  nursing theory, 30–31
  Pocketbook, sleeve
  Roy, 31
Attitudes, in critical thinking, 10
Auscultation, in physical examination, 41

B

Basic needs, Maslow's theory of, 27–29*f*
Belief patterns, on care plan, 214
Belonging needs, 28
  assessment of, 59
  nursing diagnoses for, 72*t*
Benner, P., 3, 4
Biological variations
  culture and, 16
  dominant American culture, 18
Blood pressure (BP) reading
  data analysis, 67
  physical examination, 41
Body system approach, to physical examination, 41
Breathing, assessment of, 29–30

C

Care. *See* nursing care
Care pathway, 20
Care plan, nursing, 127, 144. *See also*
    Implementation
  communication of, 161
  computer, 162
  documenting, 161–163
  examples, 152–158, 211–218, 222–230
  nursing diagnosis, 65
  nursing interventions, 134
  nursing process, 5
  outcomes in, 103
  review of, 189–194
  suggestions for writing, 162–163
  validating, 159–160
Carpenito, 79, 82
Carroll-Johnson, 30, 79
Case management. *See also* Managed care
  nursing process, 21*t*
  patient assessment, 51–54
Case management plan, and assessment,
    51–52
  comparison to nursing process, 21
Case managers, nurse, 21
Case studies
  assessment in, 57–63
    preop clinic, 57*t*
    first day surgery, 59*t*
    postop unit, 61
    home health agency, 61–63
  evaluation in, 200–205
  nursing diagnoses, 92–97
  outcome identification, 124–126
  planning, 152–158
Case study method, 56
Cephalocaudal approach, to physical
    examination, 41
Chart review, 42
Choosing
  care plan, 224
  NANDA nursing diagnosis category,
    75*t*–76*t*
Chronological age, and developmental
    task, 31–33
Clinical pathways, 20
  example of, 170–181, 218–221
  nursing interventions, 134
Cognitive-perceptual pattern, on care plan,
    213

Collaboration, nurse-physician, 81–85,
    130
Comfort promotion, NIC interventions for,
    144, 145*t*
Communication
  care plan, 223
  culture and, 14
  dominant American culture, 17
  nursing assessment, 49
  NANDA diagnosis category, 75*t*
  therapeutic, 39–40
Comorbidities, 167
Computer, standardized care plans on, 162
Conference, patient care, 161
Congestive heart failure, clinical pathway
    for, 218–221
Coping, on care plan, 214
Cost containment. *See also* managed care
    environment
  emphasis on, 5
  nursing practice, 23–24
  cost-effective, 23
Critical pathways, 20
  advantages of, 197
  examples of, 170–181, 218–221
  goals of, 151
  individualization of care, 167
  insurance companies and, 88
  managed care environment, 150–151
  patient's view of, 178*t*–181*t*
  total knee replacement, 169, 170*t*–177*t*
Critical thinkers, 194
  characteristics of, 11–12
  and nursing intervention, 144–148
Critical thinking, 8
  for assessment, 43–44
  components of, 10
  confidence in, 12
  defined, 8–9
  for diagnosis, 85
  for evaluation, 194–195
  for implementation, 165
  levels of, 11
  and nursing process, 9–10
  for outcome identification, 117–118
  for planning, 144–148
  practice exercises for, 44–48
  prompts for, in assessment, 44
Cultural differences
  and data analysis, 66

Culture, 12
  concepts of, 14–16
  defined, 13
  dominant American, 16–18
  nurses in, 12–13 (*See also* Nursing care,
    culturally competent)
  web sites for, 231–233
Culturally competent nursing care, 12–14
  assessment and, 48–51
  components of, 14
  diagnosis and, 86–87
  evaluation and, 195–197
  examples of, 50–51, 87, 149, 168, 196
  implementation and, 166, 168
  outcome identification and, 118–119
  planning and, 148–150

D
Data analysis, in nursing diagnosis, 66
Data collection, 26–48
  continuing, 164
  examples of, 57–63, 211–214, 222–225
  examination in, 40–42
  formats for, 26–33
  interview in, 35–40
  medical record review, 42
  objective data in, 33t
  observation in, 34–35
  skills for, 33–42
  subjective data, 34t
Davidhizar, R. E., 14
Developmental tasks
  and chronological age, 31–33
  major, 32t
Diagnosis, nursing, Pocketbook
  American Nurses' Association Standard
    of, 65
  activities in, 65
  at-risk, 111, 114
  at-risk/high-risk, 83
  basic human need organization,
    70–73
  care plan, 214–215, 225–230
  case management and, 20, 21t
  case studies for, 92–97
    preop clinic, 92
    first day surgery, 93
    postop unit, 94
    home health agency, 96

  collaborative problems, 81
  components of, 65
  critical thinking for, 85–86
  culturally competent care and,
    86–87
  data analysis in, 66–68
  defined, 65, 69, 78t, pocketbook
  defining characteristics for, 83–84,
    pocketbook
  examples of, 79, 82–84, 86, 92–97, 113,
    214–215, 225–229
  etiology for, 82–83
  exercises for, 90–92
  formulating, 77–80
  managed care environment, 88–90
  medical diagnoses and, 79t
  NANDA approved, 70–77, pocketbook
  NANDA categories for, 74t, 74–77
  nursing process, 2
  organized by basic human need,
    70t–77t
  organized by human response system,
    74–77
  outcomes and, 102, 113t
  outcome statement, 111–115,
    186–187
  PES format for, 82, 93–96
  possible, 79–80, 83–84
  problem identification in, 68
  process of, 65
  prompts for critical thinking, 85–86
  review of, 190–191
  risk diagnoses, 79
  in teaching plans, 138
  types of, 78–81
  validating, 84–85
  writing, 82–84
Diagnostic-related groupings (DRGs), 19
Discharge outcomes, 109–110
  achievement of, 187f
  and evaluation, 184
  patient learning in, 139–141
Discharge planning, in case management,
  52
Documentation. *See also* Data collection
  care plan of, 161–163
  nursing assessment, 42
  nursing care, 163
  responses to interventions, 183–184
DRGs. *see* Diagnostic-related groupings

E

Effectiveness, of care plan, 160
Elimination needs, nursing diagnoses for,
    69, 70t, 70–71, pocketbook
Elimination pattern, on care plan, 212
Environmental control
    culture and, 16
    in dominant American culture, 18
Environmental management, as nursing
    intervention, 128–129
Ethnocentrism, 48
Etiology, for nursing diagnosis, 82, 85
Evaluation
    activities involved in, 183, 198–199
    American Nurses' Association standard
        of, 183
    case management, 21t
    case study for, 200–205
    criterion-referenced, 185
    critical thinking for, 194–195
    culturally competent nursing care
        during, 195–197
    examples of, 186–188, 193, 200–205
    flow chart for, 199f
    managed care environment, 197–198
    nursing process, 3
    interventions, 184
    outcomes, 185–188t
    patient participation and, 185–186
    process of, 183
    review of care plan in, 189–194
Evaluative statement, writing,
    186–188t
Examination, physical, in data collection,
    40–42
Exchanging
    care plan, 223
    NANDA nursing diagnosis category,
        74t–75t
Experience
    critical thinking, 10
    problem identification, 68
Expert nurses, 3, 167
    assessment by, 25
    implementation, 165

F

Family, patient's, as intervention source,
    135
Fee for service (FFS) payment system, 19

Feeling
    on care plan, 225
    NANDA nursing diagnosis category,
        77t
Fifth vital sign, 41
Fiscal accountability, 22, 23–24
Flow chart, evaluation, 199f
Fluid needs, nursing diagnoses for, 70t
Focus area, in problem identification, 69
Functional health patterns, 30
    example of, 211–214

G

Giger, J. N., 14
Gordon, M., 30
Growth and development, 31–33

H

Health care system
    cost containment in, 5–6
    culture and, 13
Health maintenance organizations
    (HMOs), 5, 53
Health perception, on care plan, 212
Health promotion/wellness diagnoses, 78
Health promotion/wellness outcomes,
    110–111
Health teaching, in data analysis, 68
Henderson, V., 29
Hierarchy of basic human needs,
    Maslow's, 28t, 29f, 100
History, nursing
    for care plan, 212
    form for, 37
    purpose of, 35
Home health care agencies, 52
    assessment of, 61–63
    evaluation planned by, 204
    and nursing diagnosis, 96
    and patient outcomes, 126
    planning of, 157–158
Hospital policies, and outcome
    identification, 102
Human needs, 27–29
Human response system, NANDA nursing
    diagnoses based on, 74t–77t

I

Implementation. *See also* Care plan
    activities in, 159

American Nurses Association standard
of, 159
case management, 21
critical thinking for, 165
culturally competent nursing care
during, 166, 168
data collection during, 164
documentation of, 163–164
managed care environment, 166–168
nursing process, 3
process of, 159
validation of, 159–160
Intervention, nursing, 151
American Nurses Association standard
for, 127
care plan, 215–218, 225–230
categories of, 128–132
classification of, 143–144
criteria for, 135–137
defined, 127, 128
documenting responses to, 183–184
evaluating effectiveness of, 184–185
examples of, 132, 133, 136–137,
146–147, 152–158, 215–218,
225–230
independent, 131–132
nursing interventions classification
(NIC), 116, 143–145, 146–147
nurse-initiated and -ordered, 130–132
nurse-initiated and physician-ordered,
130
physician-initiated and -ordered,
129–130
problem solving and, 134–137
rationale for, 132–133, 142, 152–158,
215–218, 225–230
types of, 128–132
Interview, nursing
informal aspect of, 39
skills for, 35–40

J
Job satisfaction, and nursing process, 7
Joint Commission on Accreditation of
Healthcare Organizations
(JCAHO)
accreditation standards, 8
critical pathways, 151
patient education, 137
web site for, 231

Judgment, clinical, 9, 10. *See also* Critical
thinking

K
Kardex, nursing, 162, 163, 191
Kataoka-Yahiro, M., 10
Knee replacement, critical pathway for,
169, 170*t*–181*t*
Knowing
care plan, 225
NANDA nursing diagnosis category,
77*t*
Knowledge. *See also* Expert nurses
in critical thinking, 10
in problem identification, 68

L
Language. *See also* Communication
and culturally competent nursing care,
197
and nursing assessment, 49
Life-style changes, in data analysis, 67
Love belonging needs, 28
assessment of, 59
nursing diagnoses for, 72*t*
Lung sounds, in data analysis, 67

M
Managed care, 5
changes leading to, 18–19
defined, 19
emergence of, 5
nursing practice, 19–22
Managed care environment, 18
assessment, 51–54
evaluation in, 197–198
implementation in, 166–168
nursing diagnosis in, 88–90
outcomes in, 119–121
planning, 150–151
Maslow, A., 27–29, 100
Medicaid, web site for, 231
Medical records, in nursing
assessment, 42
Medicare, 22
access to, 53
purpose of, 19
web site for, 231
Motivation, in data analysis, 68

Moving
    care plan, 224
    NANDA nursing diagnosis category,
        76t–77

N
NANDA (see North American Nursing
    Diagnosis Association)
National Committee for Quality Assurance
    (NCQA), 5
Needs, basic human, 28t, 29f, 70t–77t, 100
Nightingale, F., 1, 3–4, 36, 129
Norms, cultural, and outcome identifica-
    tion, 119
North American Nursing Diagnosis Asso-
    ciation (NANDA), 68, 84, 116,
    144, 190
    classification system of, 30
    diagnostic categories approved by,
        74t–77t
    nursing diagnoses developed by, 69,
    Pocketbook
    web site for, 231
Notes on Nursing (Nightingale), 1, 3–4,
    36, 129
Nursing
    defined, 1
    goal of, 14
    theories, 30
Nursing Admission Assessment form, 130
Nursing assistants, 160
Nursing care
    on care plan, 160
    cost-effective, 23
    documenting, 163–164
    giving, 163–164
    Henderson's framework for, 29–30
Nursing care, culturally competent,
        (see culturally competent nursing
        care)
Nursing care plans
    middle adult, 211–221
    senior adult, 222–230
Nursing interventions
    defined, 127
    types of, 128–133
    rationale for, 132
    selecting, 134–137
Nursing Interventions Classification (NIC)
    (1996), 116, 143–145

Nursing Outcomes Classification (NOC)
    (1997), 115, 117t
Nursing practice
    elements of, 1–2
    fiscal accountability, 22–23, 24t
    managed care, 19–22
Nursing process, 2–3
    assessment in, 25
    case management plan, 21t
    critical thinking and, 9–10, 194
    defined, 2
    diagnosis in, 65
    evaluation phase of, 183
    implementation in, 159
    importance of, 5–8
    managed care environment, 18–24
    outcomes in, 99, 121
    planning in, 127, 144
    steps in, 2–3, 21
Nutritional needs, nursing diagnoses for,
        70t
Nutritional-metabolic pattern, on care
    plan, 212

O
Objective data, 33t
Observation
    F. Nightingale on, 36
    in nursing process, 3
    skills of, 34–35
Order, nursing, 127
Orem, D. E., 31
Outcome identification
    activities for, 100
    American Nurses Association standard
        of, 99
    case studies, 124–126
        preop clinic, 124
        first day surgery, 125
        postop unit, 125
        home health agency, 126
    critical thinking for, 117–118
    culturally competent care during,
        118–121
    exercises for, 121–124
    managed care environment, 119–121
    nursing diagnosis and, 113
    prompts for critical thinking
    setting priorities, 100–102

Outcomes
  care plan, 214–215, 225–230
  case management, 21*t*
  clinical outcomes, 119*t*
  classification of, 115
  components of, 104–111
  defined, 102, 103
  discharge, 109–110, 139–141, 184, 187*f*
  establishing, 102–115
  evaluation of, 185–188, 188*t*
  examples of, 107–111, 112–113, 115,
      124–126, 193, 214–215,
      225–229
  fiscal, 120
  guidelines for writing, 111–115
  health promotion/wellness, 110–111
  intermediate, 107–108, 184
  interventions and, 116*t*
  long-term, 108–109
  managed care environment, 119–121
  measurable, 114
  nursing diagnoses, 113*t*
  in nursing process, 2
  nursing-sensitive, 120
  observable, 114
  practice exercises for, 121–124
  prevention and, 102
  purpose of, 99
  realistic, 114
  review of, 191–193
Outcome statements
  components of, 104–111
  examples, 112
  need for, 103
  writing, 111–115
Oxygen needs, nursing diagnoses for, 70*t*,
      Pocketbook

P
Pain
  defined, 116
  interventions for, 116
  as nursing diagnosis, 78
  outcomes for, 113*t*, 116*t*, 117*t*
  in physical examination, 41
Pain avoidance, nursing diagnoses for,
      71*t*, Pocketbook
Pain management
  cost containment, 24
  nursing interventions for, 146*t*–147*t*

Patient
  intervention source, 135
  meaning of term, 1
  outcome achievement evaluated by,
      185–186
Patient behavior
  outcomes and, 115
  outcome statement, 104–105
Patient care team, interdisciplinary, 42
Patient learning, evaluating, 139
Patient satisfaction, 5
Patient teaching, 137–143. *See also*
      Teaching plan
Perceiving
  care plan, 224
  NANDA nursing diagnosis category,
      76*t*–77*t*
Percussion, in physical examination, 41
Performance, in outcome statement,
      105–106
PES format, for nursing diagnosis,
      82–83
Physical assessment, in data analysis, 67
Physical comfort, NIC interventions for,
      144, 145*t*
Physiological needs, in nursing assess-
      ment, 27–28, 58, 60
Physiological needs, in nursing diagnosis,
      70–71
Plan of care. *See* Care plan, nursing
Planning
  American Nurses' Association standard
      of, 127
  case management, 21
  case study for, 152–158
      preop clinic, 152
      first day surgery, 153
      postop unit, 155
      home health agency, 157
  critical thinking in, 144–148
  culturally competent nursing care
      during, 148–150
  managed care environment, 150–151
  nursing interventions, 128–147
  nursing process, 2
Practice exercises
  assessment, 54–56
  critical thinking, 44–48
  diagnosis, 90–92
  outcome identification, 121–124

Priorities, reordering of, 191
Priority setting
    culturally competent care, 101–102
    guidelines for, 100
    mutual, 101
Problem identification, in nursing
        diagnosis, 68–77
Problem list, multidisciplinary, 89
Problem solving
    vs. critical thinking, 9
    nursing interventions, 134–137
    process, 3
Professional growth, and nursing
        process, 7
Psychiatric patients, confidentiality
        and, 53

Q
Quality, emphasis on, 5
Questions, in nursing interview, 37, 38*t*

R
Readiness to learn, promotion of, 143
Reasoning, in critical thinking, 10
Reassessment, 189
Reflection, in critical thinking, 165
Reimbursement
    FFS system, 19
    managed care as system of, 20
Relating
    care plan, 223–224
    NANDA nursing diagnosis category,
        75*t*
Replanning, 191
Reproductive pattern, on care plan, 214
Resources, health care, assessment of,
        53–54
Resource utilization, 23
Respiration, assessment of, 29–30
Rest and sleep needs, nursing diagnoses
        for, 71*t*, Pocketbook
Review of nursing care plan, 189–194
Risk nursing diagnoses, 79
Role-relationship pattern, on care
        plan, 213
Roy, C., 31

S
Safety/Security
    assessment of, 58
    in care plan, 160
    need for, 28
    safety needs, in nursing diagnoses for,
        71*t*, pocketbook
    nursing interventions, 145, 147
Saylor, C., 10
Schools of nursing, and nursing
        process, 7
Scientific process, 3. *See also* Nursing
        process
Self-actualization
    assessment of, 59
    need for, 28
    nursing diagnoses for, 73*t*, pocketbook
Self-care deficit theory, Orem's, 31
Self-concept, on care plan, 213
Self-esteem
    assessment of, 59
    need for, 28
    nursing diagnoses for, 73*t*, pocketbook
Self-examination, reflective, 165
Self-perception, on care plan, 213
Sexuality/Sexual needs
    care plan, 214
    in nursing diagnoses for, 71*t*, pocket-
        book
Sleep (*See* Rest and Sleep needs)
Sleep-rest pattern, on care plan, 213
Social organization
    culture and, 15
    dominant American culture, 17–18
Social Security Act, 19
Social workers, clinical, 52, 53
Space
    culture and, 14–15
    in dominant American culture, 17
Spiritual needs, nursing diagnoses for, 72*t*,
        Pocketbook
Stachowiak, 78
Staff assignments, and nursing process, 8
Standards, nursing (ANA)
    in critical thinking, 10
    diagnosis, 65

evaluation, 183
implementation, 159
outcome identification, 99
planning, 127
Standards of Clinical Nursing Practice, 6,
    7t, 25, 65, 99, 127, 159, 183
State laws, and outcome identification,
    102
Stereotyping, 16, 48
Stimulation needs, nursing diagnoses for,
    71t, pocketbook
Stress tolerance pattern, on care
    plan, 214
Subjective data, 34t
Survival needs, and setting priorities, 101

T
Teaching plan
    components of, 142
    developing, 141
    example of, 138–139, 140–141
    problem solving and, 138
    rationale, 142
    readiness assessment in, 140
    specificity of, 139
Temperature maintenance, nursing diag-
    noses for, 70t, pocketbook
Theory, nursing
    examples of, 30–31
    problem identification, 68
Therapeutic communication, 39
Thought processes, on care plan, 225
Time
    culture and, 15–16
    dominant American culture, 18

Time frame, on outcome statement,
    106–111
Tomey, A. Marriner-, 31
TPR (temperature, pulse, respirations), in
    physical examination, 41
Tradition, 16. *See also* Cultural differ-
    ences; Culture
Transition planning, in case management,
    52
Tripp, 78
Truth seeking, 12

U
Urinary elimination
    nursing diagnoses for, 69
    problems with, 107

V
Values/valuing
    care plan, 214, 224
    NANDA nursing diagnosis category,
        75t
Variance notes, 198
Visualization, in physical examination, 41
Vital signs, in physical examination, 41

W
Web sites, 231–233
Wellness nursing diagnoses, 73, 78
Western medicine, 16, 48

NOTES

NOTES

NOTES

NOTES

NOTES

NOTES

NOTES

NOTES

NOTES

NOTES